T0314510

Comparing Clinical
Measurement Methods

Statistics in Practice

Statistics in Practice is an important international series of texts which provide detailed coverage of statistical concepts, methods and worked case studies in specific fields of investigation and study.

With sound motivation and many worked practical examples, the books show in down-to-earth terms how to select and use an appropriate range of statistical techniques in a particular practical field within each title's special topic area.

The books provide statistical support for professionals and research workers across a range of employment fields and research environments. Subject areas covered include medicine and pharmaceutics; industry, finance and commerce; public services; the earth and environmental sciences, and so on.

The books also provide support to students studying statistical courses applied to the above areas. The demand for graduates to be equipped for the work environment has led to such courses becoming increasingly prevalent at universities and colleges.

It is our aim to present judiciously chosen and well-written workbooks to meet everyday practical needs. Feedback of views from readers will be most valuable to monitor the success of this aim.

A complete list of titles in the series appears at the end of this volume.

Comparing Clinical Measurement Methods

A Practical Guide

Bendix Carstensen

*Steno Diabetes Center, Gentofte, Denmark
& Department of Biostatistics, University of Copenhagen Denmark*

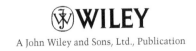

A John Wiley and Sons, Ltd., Publication

This edition first published 2010

© 2010 John Wiley & Sons Ltd

Registered office
John Wiley & Sons Ltd, The Atrium, Southern Gate, Chichester, West Sussex, PO19 8SQ, United Kingdom

For details of our global editorial offices, for customer services and for information about how to apply for permission to reuse the copyright material in this book please see our website at www.wiley.com. The right of the author to be identified as the author of this work has been asserted in accordance with the Copyright, Designs and Patents Act 1988.

Wiley also publishes its books in a variety of electronic formats. Some content that appears in print may not be available in electronic books.

Designations used by companies to distinguish their products are often claimed as trademarks. All brand names and product names used in this book are trade names, service marks, trademarks or registered trademarks of their respective owners. The publisher is not associated with any product or vendor mentioned in this book. This publication is designed to provide accurate and authoritative information in regard to the subject matter covered. It is sold on the understanding that the publisher is not engaged in rendering professional services. If professional advice or other expert assistance is required, the services of a competent professional should be sought.

Library of Congress Cataloguing-in-Publication Data

Carstensen, Bendix.
   Comparing clinical measurement methods : a practical guide / Bendix Carstensen.
      p. ; cm.
   Includes bibliographical references and index.
   ISBN 978-0-470-69423-7 (cloth)
   1.   Clinical trials – Evaluation. 2.   Clinical trials – Statistical methods.
I. Title.
   [DNLM: 1.   Clinical Medicine. 2.   Case-Control Studies. 3.   Models,
Statistical. 4.   Regression Analysis. 5.   Statistics as Topic – methods. WA
950 C321c 2010]
   R853.C55C37 2010
   610.72′4–dc22
                                                                    2010010826

A catalogue record for this book is available from the British Library.

ISBN: 978-0-470-69423-7

Typeset from the author's LaTeX source in Times by Laserwords Private Limited, Chennai, India

Contents

Acknowledgments

My workplace, Steno Diabetes Center, has throughout the last decade provided an excellent academic working environment for me and has generously given me space to pursue the statistical aspects of method comparison studies.

I am grateful to Lyle Gurrin, School of Population Health, University of Melbourne, for a long-standing collaboration on this topic and particularly for his efforts in shaping the MethComp package. My wife, Lene Theil Skovgaard, Department of Biostatistics, University of Copenhagen, has exercised a remarkable patience with this endeavor as well as an astonishingly clear insight into the problems treated. Without her assistance the book would have been less complete, with more goofs and much delayed. I dedicate this book to my children Rolf, Thor, Mira and Vega, whose never failing distrust in my intellect kept the book at a tolerable level. Any incomprehensible sections and errors in the book are therefore attributable to me alone.

1

Introduction

The classical approach to analysis of method comparison studies is the Bland–Altman plot where differences between methods are plotted against averages, leading to the limits of agreement and to verification of whether the underlying assumptions are fulfilled. This plot is merely a 45° rotation of a plot of the methods versus each other, while the limits of agreement correspond to prediction limits for the conversion between the methods.

This one-to-one correspondence between a prediction interval for the difference between two methods and the prediction of a measurement by one method given a measurement by the other is in this book carried over to an explicit modeling of data with the aim of producing conversion equations between methods.

The explicit definition of a model generating the data obtained is virtually absent in the literature. The aim of this book is to fill this gap. By explicitly defining a model for the data it is possible to discuss relevant quantities to report and their interpretation and underlying assumptions, without involving technicalities about estimation.

It is my opinion that presentation of concepts in terms of a statistical model enhances understanding, because it allows the technicalities about estimation procedures to be relegated to technical sections, and thereby allows the interpretation of models and the correspondence with practice to be discussed free of technicalities. Conversely, it is also possible to discuss estimation problems more precisely when a

Comparing Clinical Measurement Methods: A Practical Guide   Bendix Carstensen
© 2010 John Wiley & Sons, Ltd

well-defined model is specified. An explicitly defined model also makes it possible to simulate data for testing proposed measures and procedures.

The purpose of introducing explicit models is therefore not to give a formalistic derivation of all procedures, but rather to give a framework that can be used to assess the clinical relevance of the procedures proposed.

The technical sections of this book assume that the reader is familiar with standard statistical theory and practice of linear models as well as of random effects (mixed) models. However, a lack of skills should not be a major impediment to understanding the general ideas and concepts.

The core assumption in the models used in this book is that conclusions concerning the methods compared should not depend on the particular sample used for the comparison study. Taken to the extreme this is of course never true, but my point is that the particular distribution of blood glucose, say, among patients in a study should not influence conclusions regarding relationships between different methods to measure it. Samples chosen for method comparison studies should reflect the likely *range* in which comparisons are used in the future. Any attempt to make the sample used for the method comparison study representative of future *distribution* in samples where the results are applied is futile and irrelevant.

In statistical terms this means that models presented all have a systematic effect of item (individual, sample). Moreover, this point of view automatically dismisses all measures based on correlation. Hence, such measures are only mentioned briefly in this book.

The aim of the book is to give the reader access to practical tools for analyzing method comparison studies, guidance on what to report, and perhaps most importantly some guidance on how to plan comparison studies and (in the event this is not followed) hints as to what can and what cannot be inferred from such studies, and under what assumptions. An extensive treatise on general measurement problems can be found in Dunn's book [15].

The book starts with a few brief examples that highlight some of the topics in the book: (1) the simplest situation, with one measurement by each of two methods; (2) replicate measurement by each method and exchangeability; (3) linear relationship with slope different from 1; and (4) more than two methods.

The next chapter treats the situation with one measurement per individual by two methods in more depth, mentioning some of the more common methods of regression with errors in both variables. Chapter 5 treats the case where replicate measurements are taken on each individual, and gives advice on how to treat the situation with standard software.

The core of the book is Chapter 7, with the exposition of a general model that contains all the previous models as special cases. The model is expanded using transformation of data in Chapter 8.

What is *not* treated in this book are models for completely general non-linear relationships between measurement methods, except in so far as they can be transformed to the linear case. Likewise, the case of non-constant variances is also only treated in cases where data can be transformed to the constant variance case.

All graphs in this book are generated by R, and most are the result of functions specially designed to handle method comparison data collected in the package MethComp developed by Lyle Gurrin and me. The majority of the procedures in Chapters 4 and 5 can fairly easily be implemented in existing standard software. Examples of code for these methods are given in Chapter 12 for SAS, Stata and R.

When non-constant bias is introduced the underlying models become largely intractable, and the only viable method of estimation in finite (programming) time is to use either the ad-hoc procedure of alternating regressions or the BUGS machinery in one of the available implementations. The models proposed are wrapped up in the MethComp package for R.

There is a website http://www.biostat.ku.dk/~bxc/ MethComp for the MethComp package where examples and illustrative programs can be found. The website also contains links to teaching material related to this book, including practical exercises with corresponding solutions.

2

Method comparisons

When the same clinical or biochemical quantity can be measured in two ways, the natural question is to ask which one is better. This is not necessarily a meaningful question to ask, certainly not without further qualification. In this chapter the main problems and themes of method comparison treated in the book are presented through three examples.

2.1 One measurement by each method

There are, roughly speaking, two methods of measuring blood glucose: the cheap and easy method, based on a capillary blood sample taken from a simple finger prick and analyzed on a small desktop machine; and a more elaborate method, based on a venous blood sample analyzed in a proper clinical laboratory.

Figure 2.1 shows pairwise measurements of blood glucose by the two methods. It appears that the two methods do not give the same results: the venous plasma values are on average about 0.9 mmol/l greater than those from capillary blood. However, it does not appear to be easy to predict a value by one method if we have a measurement by the other, and it is not easy to tell from the data which method gives the most correct answer – in fact it is impossible. This is the characteristic of measurement *comparison* studies – there is no way to tell what the truth is, and we can only make comparisons between methods.

Comparing Clinical Measurement Methods: A Practical Guide   Bendix Carstensen
© 2010 John Wiley & Sons, Ltd

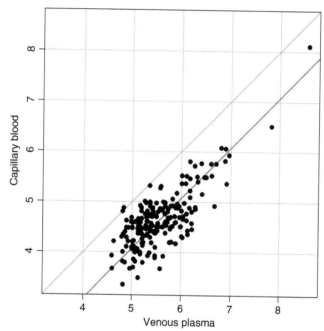

Figure 2.1   Two methods of measuring blood glucose, in mmol/l. Data are from the Addition study. These data are a subset of those published in [14], where more details are given. The line through the points is drawn at 45°, the difference from the identity line is the mean difference between methods.

With data such as those in Figure 2.1, we can get a more precise idea of the difference between methods by forming the difference between the measurements on blood and plasma for each individual. The average of these differences is about −0.9 mmol/l, so one conclusion is that capillary blood measurements are about 0.9 mmol/l smaller than plasma measurements.

Figure 2.2 shows the differences between the subject-specific blood and plasma measurements versus their corresponding averages. This allows us to see whether the difference varies systematically with the level of measurement – this is just an easier way to check whether the line through the points is parallel to the identity line. If the differences are constant, then it means that measurements by one method only differ by a constant from those by the other, i.e. that the relationship is $y_{2i} = \alpha + y_{1i}$, a line with slope 1. Here, y_{1i} is the measurement by

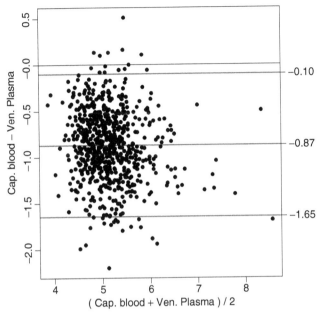

Figure 2.2   The same data as in Figure 2.1: differences versus averages and 95% prediction interval for the differences ('limits of agreement').

method 1 on individual i, and similarly for method 2. The situations where the line relating the two methods is not parallel to the identity line, and where the variation is not the same over the range of the averages, are treated later.

In Figure 2.2 we have also included lines that will approximately capture 95% of the differences – a *prediction* interval for the differences. This tells us that for 95% of the persons, the difference between a capillary blood measurement and a plasma measurement is between −1.68 and −0.17 mmol/l, and we implicitly assume that this will be the case for future patients too. This type of plot is normally termed a 'Bland–Altman plot' after the authors who first introduced it [2, 6]. They also coined the term 'limits of agreement' (LoA) for the prediction interval for the differences.

If we were to replace the plasma method by the capillary blood method then we would have to consider whether this interval is sufficiently tight around 0 from a *clinical* point of view. In this case, no one in a diabetes clinic would think so, but the important point here is that this is not *statistically* derived from data, it comes from knowledge of the practice and requirements in a diabetes clinic.

This is a characteristic of all statistical models presented in this book: they will not produce any conclusive statistic for the method comparison, but only summaries as input to clinically based decisions.

2.1.1   Prediction of one method from another

Another possibility would be to 'correct' the capillary blood values by simply adding 0.9 mmol/l to them to give values that on average match the plasma values – the predicted value of the plasma measurement given that only the capillary measurement were available. A measurement based on venous plasma would then be between −0.75 and +0.75 from this prediction with 95% probability. The bias would then be gone but we would still face the clinical question of whether the *precision* of the prediction was sufficient.

The obvious question to ask is: what is the likely value of a plasma glucose measurement (had we done one on this patient at this time), given that the capillary blood glucose measurement is 7.2 mmol/l? The straightforward answer is of course $7.2 + 0.92 = 8.1$ mmol/l and a prediction interval for this value would be of the same size as the limits of agreement, $7.2 - (-1.68, -0.17)$, i.e. from 7.4 to 8.9 mmol/l.

Note the one-to-one correspondence between limits of agreement, i.e. a prediction interval for the difference between two methods and a prediction interval for one method given a measurement by the other.

2.1.2   Why not use the correlation?

In this data set, the correlation is 0.78, not impressive, but very significantly different from 0 due to the large amount of data. However, the correlation depends largely on the selection of persons for the study; had the venous plasma values been more evenly distributed over the range from 4 to 10 mmol/l, we would have had a larger correlation, *but still the same relation between methods*. The correlation assesses the degree of relationship *in the data set*, but the aim of method comparison is to assess agreement *beyond the data set*, between the measurements in any realistically conceivable situation.

Of course the generalization from a method comparison study is limited largely to the range of measurements in the study, but the conclusions from the study should not depend on the actual distribution of measurements in any other way. In principle the conclusions should be the same with another patient sample. And this is not the case for the correlation. Chapter 10 discusses a number of other measures of association, some of which suffer from the same degree of irrelevance as the correlation.

2.1.3 A new method and a reference method

The initial presentation of the methods as 'cheap and easy' versus 'elaborate' indicates that the two methods may not be two randomly chosen methods, but rather a new candidate method and an established one, the latter possibly even a reference method ('gold standard' as it is sometimes vaguely put). In this case we could use statistical methods where we *condition* either on values obtained by the new method or by the reference method:

1. If we regress the new method on the reference method, we will learn how imprecise the new method is – the conditional mean of the new method given the reference method is the bias (relative to the reference method), and the residual variation gives the (extra) imprecision of the new method.

2. If we regress the reference method on the new method we are trying to produce a prediction of what we would have seen by the reference method for an individual with a given value of the new method.

Subsequently it will be argued that the latter approach makes assumptions that are undesirable in practical applications, and that regression of the new method on the reference method is preferable if we want to establish the relationship between the methods (i.e. predict the reference method value from a measurement by the new method).

Here it suffices to say that regression methods are derived from assumptions of the conditional distribution of the one method given the other, which in turn comes from the joint distribution, and thus implicitly assumes a particular distribution of the sample. And as future measurements cannot be guaranteed to come from this distribution, we cannot base future predictions on this.

2.2   Replicate measurements by each method

For the blood glucose data it is impossible to tell which one of the two methods is the more precise. Assessing the precision of the methods separately requires repeat measurements by each method for (at least some of) the units.

2.2.1   Exchangeable replicates: fat data

At the Steno Diabetes Center, two students, KL and SL, measured the thickness of the subcutaneous fat layer in 43 patients, with three replicate measurements by each student on each patient. The purpose of the study was to assess how well the two students agreed in the measurement of subcutaneous fat and whether the precision differed substantially between the two.

Data are shown in Figure 2.3. We see that the differences are spread nicely around 0, and that the limits of agreement are $(-0.23, 0.32)$ cm – in this case highly satisfactory (you will need to be told that it is so; the numbers do not tell us this on their own).

Since we have replicate measurements by both methods, we must decide which replicates to match when doing the plots. In Figure 2.3 we have just used the replication numbers as recorded in the file. With this data set we could have used any ordering of replicates within each item, since there is no link between replicates by one method (observer) and by the other method.

Exchangeability of replicates is a key issue in treatment of replicate measurements, as the next example illustrates.

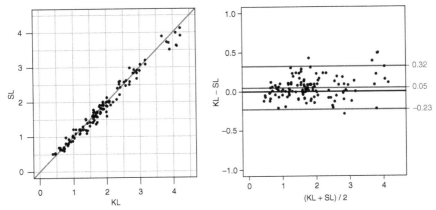

Figure 2.3   Measurements by two students of subcutaneous fat (cm) on 43 patients: scatter plot and Bland–Altman plot. Each patient is measured three times, so there are 129 points in the plot. Replicates are randomly paired for the purpose of plotting.

2.2.2   Linked replicates: oximetry data

In the Royal Children's Hospital in Melbourne, oxygen saturation (in %) of the blood of sick children were measured by two methods: CO oximetry (involving taking a proper blood sample) and pulse oximetry (a non-invasive method using light reflection on a finger or toe). The results are shown in Figure 2.4.

As opposed to the fat measurements in the previous example, the replicates are *linked* across methods, i.e. the first replicates by both methods are taken at one time, and the second replicates at slightly later time. There are random fluctuations in the actual level of oxygen saturation, but we have no reason to expect any special development from one measuring time to the next. Therefore the *pairs* of measurements are exchangeable, but the measurements are *not* exchangeable *within* methods as in the previous example. We say that the replicates are *linked* across methods.

Occasionally linked replicates occur where ordering of replicates also matters, i.e. where replicate pairs are *not* exchangeable either. This may, for example, be the case if replicates are taken at different times and some systematic effect of time is anticipated.

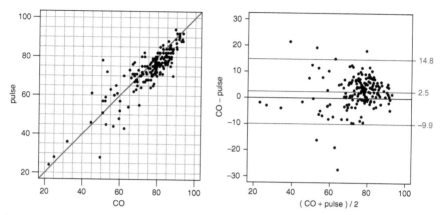

Figure 2.4   Measurements of oxygen saturation (in %) in blood by CO oximetry and by pulse oximetry. Each child is measured on three occasions, closely spaced, each time by both methods. Measurements taken at the same time by the two methods are plotted against each other, so each child contributes three points in the plot.

2.2.3   Why not use the averages of the replicates?

Sometimes the analysis is based on the averages of the replicate measurements for each person and method. This is not wrong but it addresses a different question, namely: where is the difference between the *mean* of measurements by one method and the *mean* of measurements by the other likely to be? It is rare to find a situation where this is relevant, partly because the answer depends on how many replicates the mean is based on.

Prediction of an average of a measurement by method 2 from an average of measurements by method 1 requires that the number of replicates is the same for all persons. It does not predict the difference between future *single* measurements – the limits will be too narrow.

An exception is of course the case where the *method* is *defined* as the average of, say, two measurements. In this case the analysis of single measurements would be clinically meaningless.

2.3   More than two methods

Sometimes more than two methods are compared. Bland and Altman [8] give an example of two manual readers and one automated reading of systolic blood pressure, where each person is measured by all three methods at three slightly different times, so we have linked replicates. The pairwise scatter plots and pairwise Bland–Altman plots for the three methods are shown in Figure 2.5.

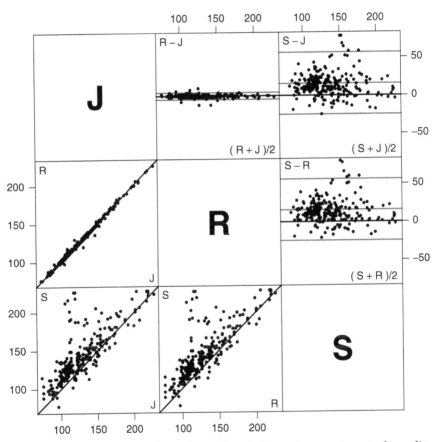

Figure 2.5   Two manual readers (J and R) and an automated reading (S) of systolic blood pressure. Each person is measured three times and so contributes three dots in each panel.

When more than two methods are compared, we can compare the methods pairwise. The pairwise comparison can be done either by analyzing data for each pair of methods, or by making a joint analysis of the entire data set allowing some of the estimates to draw on data from all methods.

The central message in Chapters 5 and 7 is that greater insight in the relationship between methods is gained by using proper statistical models to extract the information from the experimental data.

2.4   Terminology and notation

In the rest of this book the following notation will be used:

Measurement *methods* will be indexed by $m = 1, \dots, M$.

Individuals or samples will be termed *items* and indexed by $i = 1, \dots, I$.

Repeated measurements by method m on item i will be termed *replicates* and indexed by $r = 1, \dots, R_{mi}$.

When we refer to the (mean) difference between methods, we will use the term *bias*.

When discussing variance component models we will use the convention that *fixed effects* (parameters) are represented by Greek letters and *random effects* (latent variables) by Latin letters.

In most studies M will be fairly small, mostly 2 but occasionally up to 5 or 6. The number of replicates R_{mi} will also be fairly small, rarely over 5. In contrast, the number of items (persons, samples) will usually range from 20–30 (smallish) to several hundreds.

2.5   What it is all about

When measurements are taken by two methods on a group of items, then the variation between items will introduce a strong correlation between the two sets of measurements. This correlation is of course irrelevant for the method comparison, so the item effect must be removed from the method comparison.

Traditionally this is done by using the differences between the methods. Or if some more detailed analyses are needed, transform the pairwise measurements to their differences and their averages, and base analysis on these two approximately independent quantities. This is the main idea in all method comparison methods, and the rest is largely technical paraphernalia.

The formal way of getting rid of the item effects is to include a fixed effect of item in the models, which also has the advantage that it allows a more precise formulation of models describing more complex experimental plans. The rest of this book is therefore about extending the model underlying the traditional approaches.

3

How to . . .

3.1 . . .use this chapter

Reading through this book will give an overview of models to use in various method comparison situations, as well as explanations of the background and technical details about estimation procedures.

This chapter is intended to let you bypass most of this and get straight to a very brief description of what to do, what to use, and where to find more details, hopefully also including a worked example not too dissimilar from your own problem. All the descriptions in this chapter are superficial and essentially assume that you have read the rest of the book carefully. So if this is your first reading of the book, skip the rest of this chapter.

You will not be able understand much of this chapter if you do not know the sections of the book that are referred to. Therefore you can use this chapter as:

- a reminder of topics once you have read the rest of the book;

- a quick guide to the chapters where the topics you need right now are treated.

Comparing Clinical Measurement Methods: A Practical Guide   Bendix Carstensen
© 2010 John Wiley & Sons, Ltd

The chapter is subdivided by type of study and problems you may have encountered in it.

3.2   Two methods

3.2.1   Single measurements

If only one one measurement by each method is available, plot the differences versus the averages, and check whether the difference is constant and whether the variance of the difference is constant across the range of measurements.

Constant bias

If the difference is constant and its variance is also constant, then compute the limits of agreement (see Section 4.1).

Non-constant bias

If the difference between the methods is not constant across the range of measurement, then a linear relationship between methods can be estimated (see Section 4.2).

If the relationship is not linear, a suitable transformation should be found that makes the relationship linear with constant variance (see Section 4.8).

Non-constant variance

If the variance of the differences is not constant over the range of measurements, a suitable transformation should be found that makes the relationship linear with constant variance (see Section 4.8).

3.2.2   Comparing with a gold standard

If no replicate measurements are available, the assumption of one method being the 'gold standard' implies that this method measures without error. In that case, ordinary regression of the 'test' method on the 'gold standard' should be done. The resulting prediction relation, with limits for predicting the test from the standard, can also be used the other way round (see Sections 4.6 and 7.4.4).

3.2.3 Replicate measurements

If replicate measurements are available for each method the differences should be plotted versus the averages. If replicates are linked (see Chapter 5) the pairing is that of the replicates; if replicates are exchangeable, make a random pairing of replicates. Do not take averages over replicates; the variation will be underestimated if you do.

Constant bias

If the differences and their variance are constant over the range of averages, fit the relevant variance component model and report the limits of agreement based on the estimates from this (see Section 5.3).

Non-constant bias

If the difference is not constant you need to fit a non-linear variance component model as described in Chapter 7. This is not a job for standard software.

Non-constant variance

If the variance of the differences is not constant over the range of measurements, a suitable transformation should be found that makes the relationship linear (preferably with constant difference too) with constant variance (see Chapters 7 and 8).

3.3 More than two methods

If more than two methods are compared, you should decide whether they are so similar (from a substantial point of view) that it actually will make sense to compare them (see Chapter 6). The point is that you of course want results to be consistent in the sense that translation from method 1 to method 2 and translation of this result further to method 3 should give the same result as the translation directly from method 1 to method 3.

3.3.1   Single measurements

As with two methods only, you should plot differences versus averages for all pairs of methods to check the assumption of constant difference and constant variance.

Constant bias

If the differences and their variance are constant over the range of averages, you can either compute limits of agreement for all pairs of methods, or you can fit a two-way analysis of variance model and use this as the basis for reporting (see Chapter 6).

Non-constant bias

If the differences are not constant, but vary linearly with the average, the simple approach from the case of two methods (see Section 4.2) can be used for all pairs of methods. However, this does not guarantee consistent relationships between methods, so a model with linear relations between methods should be fitted, providing mutually consistent translations between methods (see Chapter 6).

Non-constant variance

As in the other cases the only feasible way to go about this is to find a transformation that makes the variance (and preferably also the mean) of the differences constant (see Chapters 7 and 8).

3.3.2   Replicate measurements

With replicate measurements on several methods you will have sufficient data to produce estimates from a proper statistical model. This will ensure estimates of consistent relationships between methods. Hence, the procedures to be used are the same as those used for the analysis of two methods with replicate measurements (see Chapter 7).

4

Two methods with a single measurement on each

This chapter treats the very simplest measurement comparison studies. Recommendations are summarized at the end of the chapter.

In Figure 4.1 there are two examples of measurements by two methods on a number of individuals. The left-hand panel shows measurements of HbA_{1c} from 38 patients by two different methods. HbA_{1c} is measured on diabetic patients to assess their long-term glucose regulation (for normal persons this is around 4–5%, and the target for diabetic patients is a value below 7%). The actual value of the measurement is the proportion of the hemoglobin that is glycosylated, hence the percentage measurement. The two methods refer to measurements performed on venous or capillary blood samples. The right-hand panel shows measurements of blood glucose concentration on 682 patients, also from either venous or capillary blood. Measurements are in mmol/l.

At first glance it seems that the agreement between the HbA_{1c} methods is much better than between the glucose methods. This is, however, a meaningless statement; what is of interest *separately* in the two cases is whether the agreement is sufficiently close for clinical ends.

Therefore, the relevant quantities are the differences between the two measurements – i.e. how far apart are they? Displaying the differences versus the average of each pair of measurements gives a picture

Comparing Clinical Measurement Methods: A Practical Guide Bendix Carstensen
© 2010 John Wiley & Sons, Ltd

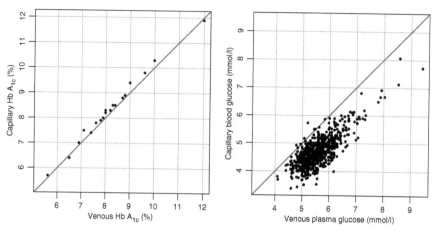

Figure 4.1   (Left) Measurements of HbA$_{1c}$ (%) based on capillary or venous blood – a subset of those published in [10]. (Right) Two methods of measuring blood glucose, from capillary or venous blood (in mmol/l). Data are based on random blood samples of patients from the Addition study, a subset of those published in [14]. Originally values are only given to the nearest 0.1 mmol/l, but here a random perturbation U(−0.04, 0.04) has been added to visually separate points.

of how large the differences are and whether they vary by the 'true' values (as, for example, represented by the average).

However, the pure scaling of the graphs, as seen in Figure 4.2, can make these displays equally deceptive. In the top panels, the HbA$_{1c}$ measurements now seem to have a very large spread, but that is due to the scaling of the y-axis (the differences). One suggestion might be to force the units to have the same physical extent on both axes, as seen in the lower panels in Figure 4.2. This is a better solution, where the physical extent of the axes normally will be determined by the range of the averages.

It is common to draw the limits of agreement, i.e. a prediction interval for the difference between measurements by the two methods.

4.1   Model for limits of agreement

The basic data are measurements y_{mi} by method m on item i. The idea behind looking at the differences is to get rid of the irrelevant

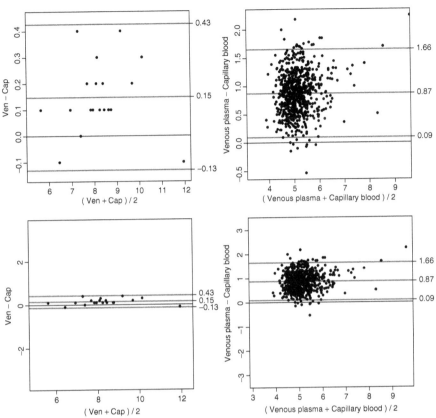

Figure 4.2   Bland–Altman plots of the same data as shown in Figure 4.1. The two top panels are drawn so that data fill the entire graph. The lower panels are drawn such that x- and y-axes have the same physical extent of the units on both scales, and such that the y-axis is symmetric around 0. The latter helps to give a graphical impression of the size of the bias and the prediction limits.

component which is the item (person, individual) effect. This implicitly assumes a model of the form

$$y_{mi} = \alpha_m + \mu_i + e_{mi}, \quad e_{mi} \sim \mathcal{N}(0, \sigma_m^2). \tag{4.1}$$

Note that we assume that the variance of the measurements is different for the two methods; it would be quite a strong assumption to assume that they were equal. But it does not mean that we can estimate the two separate variances with the data available.

This model implies that

$$d_i = y_{1i} - y_{2i} \sim \mathcal{N}(\alpha_1 - \alpha_2, \sigma_1^2 + \sigma_2^2),$$

i.e. a distribution independent of the item levels μ_i. We can estimate the quantities of interest:

$$\widehat{\alpha_1 - \alpha_2} = \bar{d}.$$

$$\widehat{\sigma_1^2 + \sigma_2^2} = \sum_i (d_i - \bar{d}.)^2/(I - 1).$$

A 95% prediction interval for the difference between a pair of measurements by the two methods on a new item is then

$$\widehat{\alpha_1 - \alpha_2} \pm 1.96 \sqrt{\widehat{\sigma_1^2 + \sigma_2^2}}$$

or

$$\bar{d}. \pm 1.96 \; \widehat{s.d.(d_i)}.$$

This is not quite correct since the estimation error of $\alpha_1 - \alpha_2$ is not taken into account. The standard error of this is $\sqrt{(\sigma_1^2 + \sigma_2^2)/I}$, and since the variance is estimated from data too, the correct limits of agreement would use a t-quantile, so the multiplying factor would be $\pm t_{0.975}(I - 1) \sqrt{(I + 1)/I}$. In practical applications it is customary to use the value 2. The term $t_{0.975}(I - 1)\sqrt{(I + 1)/I}$ is 2.08 for $I = 30$ and less than 2 if $I > 85$ (and converges to 1.96 for $I \rightarrow \infty$; for $I > 668$ it rounds to 1.96). Thus the pragmatic rule of using 2 gives a slight overestimate of the limits for large studies and an underestimate for smaller studies (however, relying on an assumption of a normal distribution of measurements).

4.1.1   Prediction between methods

The limits of agreement form a prediction interval for the difference between measurements by the two methods on the same item.

This is in one-to-one correspondence with a prediction interval for a measurement by method 2 given a measurement by method 1. The limits of agreement rely on estimates of the parameters $\alpha_1 - \alpha_2$ and $\sigma_1^2 + \sigma_2^2$ from model (4.1).

Using the same model to predict a measurement by method 2 on a new item, 0, say, given a measurement by method 1, y_{10}, say, goes a follows. The mean of the measurement by method 1 is $\alpha_1 + \mu_0$, and the mean of measurement to be predicted is $\alpha_2 + \mu_0 = (\alpha_2 - \alpha_1) + \alpha_1 + \mu_0$. The only piece of information on the new item is y_{10}, so this is the best estimate of $\alpha_1 + \mu_0$, and since we have an estimate of $\alpha_2 - \alpha_1$ from the calibration data set, the predicted mean is just the sum of these two estimates:

$$\hat{y}_{20} = \widehat{\alpha_2 - \alpha_1} + \widehat{\alpha_1 + \mu_0} = \bar{d}. + y_{10}.$$

The variance of this sum of two independent quantities is the sum of the variances:

$$\mathrm{var}(\hat{y}_{20}) = (\sigma_1^2 + \sigma_2^2)/I + \sigma_1^2.$$

Now, since we want a *prediction* interval for y_{20}, we want the prediction variance, which is the sum of the variance of the estimated mean (as above) plus the variance of the new observation y_2, which is σ_2^2:

$$\mathrm{var}(y_{20}) = (\sigma_1^2 + \sigma_2^2)/I + \sigma_1^2 + \sigma_2^2 = (\sigma_1^2 + \sigma_2^2)(I + 1)/I.$$

So a 95% prediction interval for y_{20} is

$$y_{10} \pm 1.96\sqrt{(I + 1)/I} \times \mathrm{s.d.}(d_i).$$

As for the limits of agreement, the correct expression for the multiplier would be $t_{0.975}(I - 1)\sqrt{(I + 1)/I}$, but 2 is commonly used.

Thus we see there is a one-to-one correspondence between the limits of agreement and a prediction interval for a measurement by one method given one by the other. The Bland–Altman plot is just a 45° rotation of the plot of the measurements by the two methods. The rotated plot of the limits of agreement simply corresponds to the prediction limits, which moreover has the property that they can be used both ways. This is illustrated in Figure 4.3.

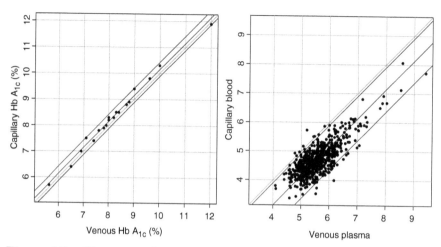

Figure 4.3   The same plots as in Figure 4.1, but with prediction limits drawn. The plots are really just 45° rotations of the Bland–Altman plots in the bottom panels of Figure 4.2.

4.1.2   The correlation of the difference and the average

It has been pointed out [7] that when we draw a Bland–Altman plot, the difference and the average of the two measurements are correlated. Now, let the *marginal variances* be $\mathrm{var}(y_{1i}) = \tau_1^2$ and $\mathrm{var}(y_{2i}) = \tau_2^2$; then

$$\mathrm{cov}\,(y_{1i} - y_{2i}, (y_{1i} + y_{2i})/2) = \frac{\tau_1^2 - \tau_2^2}{2},$$

$$\mathrm{corr}\,(y_{1i} - y_{2i}, (y_{1i} + y_{2i})/2) = \frac{\tau_1^2 - \tau_2^2}{\tau_1^2 + \tau_2^2}.$$

Therefore, if we suspect, for example, that $\tau_2 \gg \tau_1$ we should expect a negative slope in the points on the Bland–Altman plot. In most practical situations this effect is, however, rather small, because the computation of the correlation above refers to the *marginal* distributions of y_1 and y_2. In model (4.1) the marginal variances are $\tau_m^2 = \mathrm{var}(\mu_i) + \sigma_m^2$, and hence the correlation is

$$\frac{\tau_1^2 - \tau_2^2}{\tau_1^2 + \tau_2^2} = \frac{\sigma_1^2 - \sigma_2^2}{2\mathrm{var}(\mu_i) + \sigma_1^2 + \sigma_2^2}.$$

Note that this is heavily dependent on the way the items (i.e. the μ_is) are chosen for the particular experiment. Hence it depends *both* on characteristics of the methods *and* characteristics of the design, the latter being alien to the method comparison.

In realistic circumstances, one would normally choose a range for the true values (the μ_is) that is wide compared to the measurement error, i.e. so that $\text{var}(\mu_i) \gg \sigma_m$, $m = 1, 2$. If the empirical variance of the 'true' values in a sample were of the same order of magnitude as the measurement errors, we would have methods that were barely capable of distinguishing any items in the sample. This would mean that the study was either badly designed (too narrow a range of the true values) or that (at least) one of the methods was so imprecise that it would be clinically useless. Neither situation is likely to occur in real applications, so the correlation between differences and averages is rarely of any practical importance.

4.2   Non-constant difference between methods

If it is observed that the assumption of constant difference between methods is violated, i.e. if there is a clear slope in the Bland–Altman plot, it has been suggested that one might regress the differences on the averages and use the regression to construct prediction intervals for the difference between two future measurements. In order to get this on a proper formal footing we set up a model for the measurements, and from that derive a model for the relationship between differences and averages, and subsequently use the estimates from the regression of differences on averages to get back to the quantities of interest.

We use a model where measurements by each of the methods are related linearly to a 'true' value, μ_i for each item – basically extending the model (4.1) with a linear term:

$$
\begin{aligned}
y_{1i} &= \alpha_1 + \beta_1 \mu_i + e_{1i}, \quad e_{1i} \sim \mathcal{N}(0, \sigma_1^2), \\
y_{2i} &= \alpha_2 + \beta_2 \mu_i + e_{2i}, \quad e_{2i} \sim \mathcal{N}(0, \sigma_2^2).
\end{aligned}
\tag{4.2}
$$

Model (4.1) is the sub-model of (4.2) where $\beta_1 = \beta_2 = 1$. Model (4.2) is attractive because it is symmetric in the methods; exchanging the methods merely means a change in sign of the regression coefficients, whereas regression of method 1 on method 2 would give a different relation than regression the other way round. We would like the algorithms to be symmetric in the methods we are comparing. It would, for example, be an attractive feature if corresponding prediction intervals between methods looked the same on a plot regardless of the direction of use, as was the case for the simple model (4.1).

Given a single observation of y_1 for a new item (called '0'), y_{10}, this is the only piece of data available for estimation of the 'true' mean μ_0 for this item. Using the model, the prediction of y_{20} from y_{10} is derived by isolating μ_0 from the first equation and then inserting this in the second. This gives

$$y_{2|1} = \alpha_2 + \beta_2\mu_0 + e_{20} = \left(\alpha_2 - \alpha_1\frac{\beta_2}{\beta_1}\right) + \frac{\beta_2}{\beta_1}y_1 + \frac{\beta_2}{\beta_1}e_{10} + e_{20}$$

$$(4.3)$$

$$= \alpha_{2|1} + \beta_{2|1}y_{10} + e_{2|1} \quad e_{2|1} \sim \mathcal{N}(0, \sigma_{2|1}^2).$$

The parameters of interest for prediction between the two methods of measurement can now be expressed in terms of the parameters of the model:

$$\text{intercept,} \quad \alpha_{2|1} = \alpha_2 - \alpha_1\frac{\beta_2}{\beta_1};$$

$$\text{slope,} \quad \beta_{2|1} = \frac{\beta_2}{\beta_1}; \qquad (4.4)$$

$$\text{prediction variance,} \quad \sigma_{2|1}^2 = \left(\frac{\beta_2}{\beta_1}\right)^2\sigma_1^2 + \sigma_2^2.$$

Predicting the other way round is symmetric to this,[1]

In order to obtain estimates of the parameters of interest, we consider the model induced by (4.2) for the differences $D_i = y_{1i} - y_{2i}$

---

[1] Or, as a mathematician would put it, '... is obtained by permutation of the method indices'.

and the averages $A_i = (y_{1i} + y_{2i})/2$:

$$D_i = (\alpha_1 - \alpha_2) + (\beta_1 - \beta_2)\mu_i + e_{1i} - e_{2i};$$
$$A_i = (\alpha_1 + \alpha_2)/2 + (\beta_1 + \beta_2)\mu_i/2 + (e_{1i} + e_{2i})/2.$$

In parallel to the previous derivation, the relationship between D_i and A_i can be expressed by isolating μ_i from the expression for A_i,

$$\mu_i = [2A_i - (\alpha_1 + \alpha_2) - (e_{1i} + e_{2i})]/(\beta_1 + \beta_2),$$

and inserting this in the expression for D_i,

$$D_i = (\alpha_1 - \alpha_2) + \frac{\beta_1 - \beta_2}{\beta_1 + \beta_2}[2A_i - (\alpha_1 + \alpha_2) - (e_{1i} + e_{2i})] + e_{1i} - e_{2i}$$

$$= (\alpha_1 - \alpha_2) - (\alpha_1 + \alpha_2)\frac{\beta_1 - \beta_2}{\beta_1 + \beta_2}$$

$$+ \frac{\beta_1 - \beta_2}{\beta_1 + \beta_2}2A_i$$

$$+ e_{1i}\left(1 - \frac{\beta_1 - \beta_2}{\beta_1 + \beta_2}\right) - e_{2i}\left(1 + \frac{\beta_1 - \beta_2}{\beta_1 + \beta_2}\right)$$

This suggests fitting a linear regression of the differences on the averages,

$$D_i = a + bA_i + e_i, \qquad e_i \sim \mathcal{N}(0, \tau^2), \qquad (4.5)$$

and then, based on estimates of a, b and τ^2 from this model, computing the parameters of interest. The relationships are (using the relations from (4.4)):

$$
\left.
\begin{aligned}
a &= (\alpha_1 - \alpha_2) - (\alpha_1 + \alpha_2)\frac{\beta_1 - \beta_2}{\beta_1 + \beta_2} \\
b &= 2\frac{\beta_1 - \beta_2}{\beta_1 + \beta_2} \\
\tau^2 &= \left(\frac{2\beta_1}{\beta_1 + \beta_2}\right)^2 \left(\frac{\beta_2^2}{\beta_1^2}\sigma_1^2 + \sigma_2^2\right)
\end{aligned}
\right\}
\Leftrightarrow
\left\{
\begin{aligned}
\alpha_{2|1} &= \frac{-a}{1 + b/2} \\
\beta_{2|1} &= \frac{1 - b/2}{1 + b/2} \\
\sigma_{2|1} &= \frac{\tau}{(1 + b/2)}
\end{aligned}
\right.
\qquad (4.6)
$$

The formulae for predicting from method 2 to method 1 follow from symmetry; if we instead regressed the opposite differences $y_2 - y_1$ on the sums, we would just get opposite values of a and b; τ would remain unchanged.

Note that the two prediction standard deviations are related to the slope of the prediction line as

$$\frac{\sigma_{2|1}}{\sigma_{1|2}} = \frac{\tau}{1 + b/2} \bigg/ \frac{\tau}{1 - b/2} = \frac{1 - b/2}{1 + b/2} = \beta_{2|1}. \tag{4.7}$$

This implies that a graph with the line converting method 1 to method 2, $y_2 = \alpha_{2|1} + \beta_{2|1}y_1$, and the corresponding prediction limits can be used for prediction the other way too, i.e. the prediction limit lines will be usable both ways.

So from a simple linear regression of differences on averages we can compute the parameters needed to provide a prediction equation from one method to another.

However, a vital assumption behind this approach is carried over from the simple model with constant bias. If differences and sums of measurements are to be meaningful the measurements must necessarily be on the same scale; there is an underlying assumption that the two methods measure on the same scale.

4.3   A worked example

Blood glucose measurements were made on 46 persons, 120 minutes after a 75 g glucose challenge, measured in either venous plasma or capillary blood. These data are part of the glucose data set that is included in the MethComp package for R, and which is analyzed in [12].

A plot of the differences versus the averages show a clear linear trend; the slope is 0.33 with a standard error of 0.09, highly significant. The limits of agreement are quite wide; $0.37 \pm 2 \times 1.23 = (-2.09, 2.83)$, i.e. a width of about 2.5 mmol/l on either side. The regression of the differences on the averages gives a residual standard deviation of 1.08, so there is definitely room for improvement of the prediction limits.

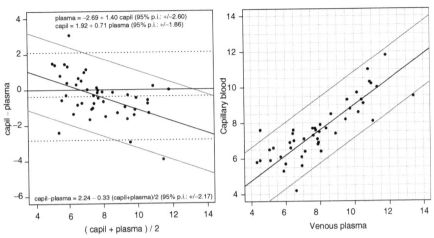

Figure 4.4   Bland–Altman plot and prediction plot for blood glucose measurements by capillary (whole) blood and venous plasma.

The left-hand panel in Figure 4.4 shows the limits of agreement as well as the prediction limits from the regression of the difference on the averages. The formulae for the derived conversion equations are also given in the plot. The right-hand panel in Figure 4.4 shows the relation between capillary blood and venous plasma as derived from the regression (rotating the left-hand plot 45° counterclockwise). Only one set of prediction limits is needed in the plot; they are applicable both ways as the prediction standard deviations differ by a factor equal to the slope of the conversion.

4.4   What really goes on

4.4.1   Scaling

Model (4.2) is qualitatively different from model (4.1), because the βs introduce a *scaling* between the methods. If all measurements by method 2 were multiplied by the same factor, the model would still be the same; the parameters α_2, β_2 and σ_2 would just be multiplied by this factor, everything else would be unchanged.

So, strictly speaking, the methods measure on different scales, and hence it is meaningless to form differences or averages between them.

Having said that, in practice it may very well still be meaningful to accept that the measurements are on the same scale and use the approach of regressing differences on averages.

4.4.2   Independence

In a regression model we assume that the error terms are independent of the regressors. But under model (4.2) the error terms in the regression (4.5) are not independent of the explanatory variable (i.e. the averages):

$$
\mathrm{cov}(A_i, e_i) = \mathrm{cov}\left[\frac{e_{1i} + e_{2i}}{2}, e_{1i}\left(1 - \frac{\beta_1 - \beta_2}{\beta_1 + \beta_2}\right) - e_{2i}\left(1 + \frac{\beta_1 - \beta_2}{\beta_1 + \beta_2}\right)\right]
$$

$$
= \frac{1}{2}\left\{\sigma_1^2 - \sigma_2^2 - \frac{\beta_1 - \beta_2}{\beta_1 + \beta_2}(\sigma_1^2 + \sigma_2^2)\right\}
$$

(see [12]). This is 0 if $\beta_{2|1} = \beta_2/\beta_1 = \sigma_2^2/\sigma_1^2$, i.e. if the slope relating the means equals the ratio of the residual variances – a condition that does not lend itself to immediate clinical interpretation. It is of course also 0 if $\sigma_1 = \sigma_2$ and $\beta_1 = \beta_2$, i.e. if the difference between the methods is constant and the residual standard deviations are equal. In which case the regression would be superfluous.

In practice this correlation is not so large that it actually matters much; it merely highlights the trick in converting the original pairs of measurements to the pairs of differences and averages. Under model (4.2) with similar βs it is a transformation to approximately independent observations.

4.4.3   Actual behavior

In [11] it is shown by means of simulation that the procedure outlined above actually performs reasonably well in terms of producing prediction intervals if the value of $\beta_{2|1}$ is not too far from 1 (i.e. in the range 0.8–1.25). This method can be recommended in situations where only one measurement per method is available, and where it can be assumed that the two methods measure on the same scale.

4.5 Other regression methods for non-constant bias

4.5.1 Why ordinary regression fails

There are basically two reasons why ordinary regression fails in method comparison studies: a formal statistical one and a conceptual one.

Statistical failure

The model underlying the ordinary regression model treats the measurement methods asymmetrically; it can be seen as a model that assumes that measurements by one method are error-free, which is clearly wrong.

In a traditional regression model it is implicitly assumed that the error terms are independent of the explanatory variable. If the traditional regression procedure of y_2 on y_1 is used on data generated under model (4.2), this assumption is violated, because the model establishes a relationship between y_2 and y_1 as shown in equation (4.3),

$$y_2 = \left(\alpha_2 - \alpha_1 \frac{\beta_2}{\beta_1}\right) + \left(\frac{\beta_2}{\beta_1}\right) y_1 + \left(\frac{\beta_2}{\beta_1} e_{1i} + e_{2i}\right),$$

but y_1 (the regression variable) is not independent of the error term $\frac{\beta_2}{\beta_1} e_{1i} + e_{2i}$; in model (4.2) the correlation is $1/\sqrt{2} = 0.71$.

The point of basing inference on regression of differences on averages is that the averages are approximately uncorrelated with the error terms if the slope (β_2/β_1) is not too different from 1. So the regression of differences on averages is wrong on this account too, but quantitatively much less so.

Conceptual failure

Ordinary regression of y_2 on y_1 is essentially modeling the conditional expectation of y_2 *given* y_1, i.e. a conditional distribution. While it may be argued that this does not imply assumptions about the *joint* distribution of (y_2, y_1), the actual procedure used is based on the theory for the two-dimensional normal distribution. Thus, there is an assumption about the marginal distribution of y_1, used in the prediction formula from ordinary regression.

Loosely speaking, the mechanics is that if y_1 is large it is taken as being an observation where the random error is large (positive), and hence the prediction should be made 'as if' the 'true' y_1 were a bit smaller. Hence the well-known regression to the mean.

But in method comparison studies where the focus is to say something generalizable *beyond* a particular data set, applicable to a different population of items, it is irrelevant to involve assumptions about the particular distribution of the calibration sample.

4.5.2   Deming regression

Deming regression incorporates errors in both variables. Specifically, it is restricted maximum likelihood estimation in model (4.2). Formally, this is not possible, because the model is not identifiable, not even with a restriction such as $\alpha_1 = 0$, $\beta_1 = 1$; without replicate measurements the likelihood will have two (infinite) maxima corresponding to $\sigma_1 = 0$ and $\sigma_2 = 0$, respectively. The two maxima correspond to the ordinary linear regressions of y_2 on y_1 and vice versa.

However, the model *is* identifiable if the ratio $\lambda = \sigma_2^2/\sigma_1^2$ is known; then the estimates in model (4.2) are

$$\alpha_1 = 0, \qquad \hat{\alpha}_2 = \overline{y_2} - \overline{y_1}\hat{\beta}_2,$$

$$\beta_1 = 1, \qquad \hat{\beta}_2 = \frac{\text{SSD}_2 - \lambda\text{SSD}_1 + \sqrt{(\text{SSD}_2 - \lambda\text{SSD}_1)^2 + 4\lambda\text{SPD}^2}}{2\text{SPD}},$$

$$\hat{\mu}_i = \frac{\lambda y_{1i} + \hat{\beta}(y_{2i} - \hat{\alpha})}{\lambda + \hat{\beta}^2},$$

$$\hat{\sigma} = \sqrt{\frac{\lambda \sum_{i=1}^{n}(y_{1i} - \hat{\mu}_i)^2 + \sum_{i=1}^{n}(y_{2i} - \hat{\alpha} - \hat{\beta}\hat{\mu}_i)^2}{2\lambda(n - 2)}}.$$

Here, $\text{SSD}_m = \sum_i (y_{mi} - \bar{y}_{m\cdot})^2$, $m = 1, 2$, and $\text{SPD} = \sum_i (y_{1i} - \bar{y}_{1\cdot})(y_{2i} - \bar{y}_{2\cdot})$.

These formulae are implemented in the `Deming` function in the `MethComp` package, which also contains a document with a detailed derivation of the formulae.

Deming regression is of limited practical use because it requires a priori knowledge of the ratio of the variances, which is rarely available without replicate measurements by each method. And in that case the model is actually identifiable (see Section 7) and hence Deming regression is superfluous.

Deming regression can be used as a second step in the case where replicate measurements are made. The first step is to use the replicates to estimate the method-specific residual variances, and the second is Deming regression using the mean of replicates to estimate the relationship between methods.

4.6   Comparison with a gold standard

The details of the Deming regression give a hint as to what to do in the situation where one of two methods compared is a gold standard assumed to be without error. In terms of model (4.2), if the reference method is method 1, an assumption of no error amounts to assuming that $\sigma_1 = 0$, in which case the Deming regression degenerates to regression of y_2 on y_1.

Thus, in this case, where we want to predict what a measurement by the gold standard would have been, given only a measurement by the imperfect method 2, we should use the 'usual' prediction limits for $y_{2|1}$ the other way round. This is, in other words, the limiting scenario of comparing two methods where one has a much larger residual variance than the other. However, this is not the entire story; when more sources of variation are considered, this may be an oversimplification (cf. Section 7.4.4).

4.7   Non-constant variance

One of the central assumptions in the traditional analysis of measurement comparison studies is homoscedasticity, i.e. that the variance of measurements is the same across the range of measurement values.

In the application of results it is also assumed that the variance is the same regardless of the (new, unknown) item analyzed. The background for this is that most particular assumptions of variance dependency would render the prediction possibilities void in practice.

The assumption of constant variance is normally checked by visual inspection of the Bland–Altman plot. A formal test of increasing or decreasing variance by the level of measurement can be obtained by first regressing the differences on the averages and then regressing the absolute residuals from this on the averages [1].

In Section 4.2 we saw that the prediction limits linking two methods were applicable both ways, because the ratio of the prediction standard deviations was equal to the slope of the prediction line (cf. Figure 4.4 and formula (4.7)). This is not possible with a model where the standard deviation increases linearly with the measurements.

If the standard deviation increases linearly by the measurement value with slope Δ and the conversion line has slope β, we will get prediction limits that are straight lines with slopes $\beta + 2\Delta$ and $\beta - 2\Delta$, respectively. Then the horizontal distances between each of these two lines and the conversion line are not the same. If the vertical distance at some point between the conversion line and the two prediction limits is k say (see Figure 4.5), the vertical distance between the upper line (with slope $\beta + 2\Delta$) and the central line is $k/(\beta + 2\Delta)$, but the distance between the conversion line and the lower line with slope $\beta - 2\Delta$ is $k/(\beta - 2\Delta)$. So linearly diverging prediction limits can never be usable both ways, as in the case with constant prediction standard deviations.

In practice, the only feasible way to arrive at prediction limits that are usable both ways is to find a transformation of data that makes the standard deviation constant over the relevant range. A discussion of transformations and examples can be found in Chapter 8.

4.7.1   Regression approach

Bland & Altman [8] proposed a simple approach to estimation of an increasing standard deviation of measurements in the case with one measurement by each method per item:

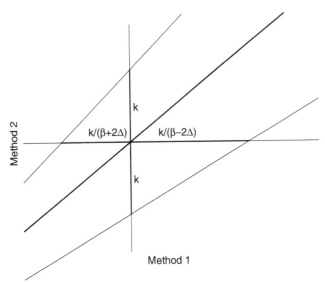

*Figure 4.5   Illustration of the impossibility of identical linear predic-
tion limits when the standard deviation is linearly increasing. The three
lines have slope $\beta + 2\Delta$, β and $\beta - 2\Delta$, respectively.*

1. Regress differences on averages and compute the residuals.

2. Regress the absolute values of the residuals on the averages to
   estimate how the standard deviation depends on the average.

3. Use these two regressions to generate prediction limits for the
   differences as a function of the averages.

The mechanics in this approach is that if residuals are normally distributed with mean 0 and standard deviation σ, the absolute residuals
follow a half-normal distribution,[2] which has mean $\sigma\sqrt{2/\pi}$. Hence the
fitted values from the regression of the absolute values on the averages
can just be multiplied by $\sqrt{\pi/2}$ to give the expected standard deviation
of the difference as function of the average of the two measurements.

---

[2] The expectation in a half-normal distribution with standard deviation 1 is

$$E(X) = \int_0^\infty (2x/\sqrt{2\pi}) \exp(-x^2/2)\mathrm{d}x = -(2/\sqrt{2\pi})\left[\exp(-x^2/2)\right]_0^\infty$$

$$= -(2/\sqrt{2\pi})(0 - 1) = \sqrt{2/\pi}.$$

The regression of the absolute residuals on the averages can be used to construct limits of agreement; these limits of agreement will refer to prediction limits for the difference between measurements by the two methods given their average. This is clearly useful from a clinical point of view when the desire is to evaluate whether one method may be substituted for the other (and vice versa). However, if the aim is to produce a prediction of the likely measurement by method 2 given a measurement by method 1, some modification is needed.

Model for increasing standard deviation

Recall from Section 4.2 that when the relation between differences $D = y_1 - y_2$ and averages $A = (y_1 + y_2)/2$ is $D_i = a + bA_i + e_i$, the prediction of y_2 from y_1 comes to

$$y_{2|1} = \frac{-a}{1 + b/2} + \frac{1 - b/2}{1 + b/2} y_1 \pm 2 \times \frac{\tau}{1 + b/2}. \qquad (4.8)$$

Now suppose that the standard deviation τ as a function of the differences is estimated to be $\tau = \alpha + \beta A$. We could then use y_1 as a surrogate of A to compute τ as a function of A, but it would be more natural to use an estimate of the average based on y_1:

$$\hat{A} = (y_1 + y_{2|1})/2 = \left(y_1 + \frac{-a}{1 + b/2} + \frac{1 - b/2}{1 + b/2} y_1 \right) \Big/ 2 = \frac{y_1 - a/2}{1 + b/2}.$$

Inserting this in $\tau = \alpha + \beta \hat{A}$ and this in turn in the expression for the prediction limits given in (4.8) gives

$$y_{2|1} = \frac{-a}{1 + b/2} + \frac{1 - b/2}{1 + b/2} y_1 \pm 2$$
$$\times \left(\frac{\alpha(1 + b/2) - a/2}{(1 + b/2)^2} + y_1 \frac{\beta}{(1 + b/2)^2} \right). \qquad (4.9)$$

In this expression, a, b are the coefficients from regression of $D = y_1 - y_2$ on $A = (y_1 + y_2)/2$, and α, β the coefficients in the linear relation of the standard deviations to the average, i.e. obtained from the coefficients from the regression of the absolute residuals on the average by multiplication by $\sqrt{\pi/2}$.

Had we formed the differences the other way round, we would have gotten the opposite coefficients from the regression of differences on averages but the same absolute residuals, so the prediction the other way round would be (still referring to the parameters from the regression of $D = y_1 - y_2$ on $A = (y_1 + y_2)/2$)

$$y_{1|2} = \frac{a}{1 - b/2} + \frac{1 + b/2}{1 - b/2} y_2 \pm 2$$
$$\times \left(\frac{\alpha(1 - b/2) + a/2}{(1 - b/2)^2} + y_2 \frac{\beta}{(1 - b/2)^2} \right). \quad (4.10)$$

Thus drawing the prediction of means in a coordinate system with y_2 versus y_1 gives the same line for the two predictions. But the limits for $y_{2|1}$ have slopes

$$\frac{1 - b/2}{1 + b/2} - 2\frac{\beta}{(1 + b/2)^2} \quad \text{and} \quad \frac{1 - b/2}{1 + b/2} + 2\frac{\beta}{(1 + b/2)^2},$$

whereas the limits for $y_{1|2}$ have slopes

$$\frac{1 + b/2}{1 - b/2} - 2\frac{\beta}{(1 - b/2)^2} \quad \text{and} \quad \frac{1 + b/2}{1 - b/2} + 2\frac{\beta}{(1 - b/2)^2},$$

which are not the inverse of the other ones, and hence these two sets of limits cannot be identical if plotted in the same coordinate system.

Thus the regression of absolute residuals on averages does not immediately translate into a symmetric conversion procedure.

Using the limits of agreement directly

A more blunt approach would be to take the limits of agreement derived from the regression of the absolute residuals on the averages (A_i) and obtain (using the approach mentioned above)

$$\tau = \alpha + \beta A.$$

Assuming the mean relationship between D and A to be $D = a + bA$, the prediction limits for D would then be

$$D = a \pm 2\alpha + (b \pm 2\beta)A.$$

If we just transform these three lines to the (y_1, y_2) coordinate system, we get prediction limits for $y_1|y_2$:

$$
\begin{aligned}
y_i &= \frac{a \pm 2\alpha}{1 - (b \pm 2\beta)/2} + \frac{1 + (b \pm 2\beta)/2}{1 - (b \pm 2\beta)/2} \times y_2 \\
&= \frac{a \pm 2\alpha}{1 - (b/2 \pm \beta)} + \frac{1 + (b/2 \pm \beta)}{1 - (b/2 \pm \beta)} \times y_2.
\end{aligned}
\tag{4.11}
$$

Since this is just a transformation of the lines derived for the relationship between (A, D), the corresponding derivation for $y_2|y_1$ will give the same lines, i.e. the same relation between y_1 and y_2.

However, this is an entirely ad-hoc procedure that suffers from the same shortcomings as the similar method with constant standard deviation mentioned in Section 4.2 and discussed in Section 4.4.

4.7.2   A worked example

Table 2 in [8] gives a data set with plasma volume as a percentage of normal. The data are shown in Figures 4.6, 4.7 and 4.8, and they are available as a data frame in the `MethComp` package:

```
> library( MethComp )
> data( plvol )
> str( plvol )

'data.frame':        198 obs. of  3 variables:
 $ meth: Factor w/ 2 levels "Hurley","Nadler": 2 2 2 2 2 2 2 2 2 2 ...
 $ item: num  1 2 3 4 5 6 7 8 9 10 ...
 $ y   : num  56.9 63.2 65.5 73.6 74.1 77.1 77.3 77.5 77.8 78.9 ...

> plvol$meth <- relevel( plvol$meth, 2 )
> plvol <- Meth( plvol )

The following variables from the data frame
"plvol" are used as the Meth variables:
meth: meth
item: item
   y: y
        #Replicates
```

```
Method            1 #Items #Obs: 198 Values:  min   med    max
  Nadler         99      99         99          56.9 99.0 133.2
  Hurley         99      99         99          52.9 90.4 121.6

> plw <- to.wide( plvol )
```

First we generate a Bland–Altman plot, where we plot both the traditional limits of agreement with the prediction limits for the differences as a function of the averages. These are produced by regressing the differences on the averages, and the drawing the regression line and the lines parallel to this at a distance of twice the residual standard deviation. This is done by using the facilities of the BA.plot function, which automatically generates these lines. It also generates the limits of agreement based on the model with constant difference, which we add subsequently:

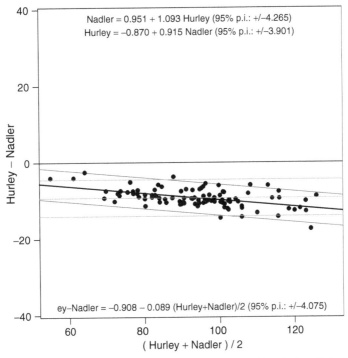

Figure 4.6   The plasma volume data from table 2 in [8]: Bland–Altman plot with limits of agreement and prediction limits based on the regression of differences on averages.

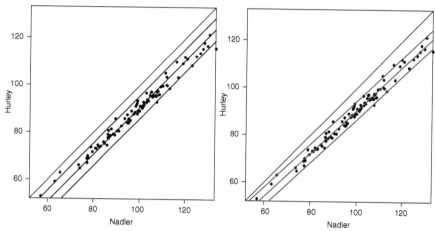

Figure 4.7 The plasma volume data from table 2 in [8]. Left: Prediction plot assuming constant difference (limits of agreement). Right: Prediction plot based on the regression of differences on averages assuming constant variance.

```
> par(mar=c(3,3,1,1), mgp=c(3,1,0)/1.6, las=1 )
> plvol.BA <- BA.plot( plvol, reg.line=3, limx=c(55,130), eqax=T, lwd=2 )

Limits of agreement:
Hurley - Nadler      2.5% limit       97.5% limit          SD(diff)
      -9.262626     -14.068455        -4.456798            2.402914

Hurley-Nadler = -0.908 - 0.089 (Hurley+Nadler)/2 (95% p.i.: +/-4.075)
  res.sd = 2.037    se(beta) = 0.014 , P = 0.0000

Nadler = 0.951 + 1.093 Hurley (95% p.i.: +/-4.265)
Hurley = -0.870 + 0.915 Nadler (95% p.i.: +/-3.901)

> abline( h=plvol.BA$LoA[1:3], col=gray(0.5) )
```

The limits of agreement can be rotated to represent prediction limits under the model with constant difference between the methods, as is shown in the next panel. The lines plotted are merely lines with slope 1, offset vertically by the mean difference and the limits of agreement:

```
> par(mar=c(3,3,1,1), mgp=c(3,1,0)/1.6, las=1 )
> with( plw, plot(Hurley ~ Nadler, pch=16, xlim=c(55,130), ylim=c(55,130)) )
> abline(0,1)
> abline(plvol.BA$LoA[1],1,lwd=2,col="blue")
> abline(plvol.BA$LoA[2],1,lwd=2,col="blue")
> abline(plvol.BA$LoA[3],1,lwd=2,col="blue")
> with( plw, points( Hurley ~ Nadler, pch=16 ) )
> box()
```

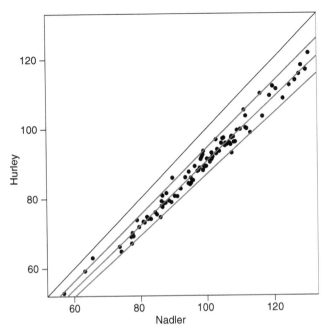

Figure 4.8   The plasma volume data from table 2 in [8]: Prediction plot accommodating increasing standard deviation, using the regression of absolute residuals on the averages.

We can do the same with the lines based on the regression of the differences on the averages, as is seen in the right panel in Figure 4.7. The BA.plot function automatically computes the regression of differences on averages and converts it to the corresponding two relations between the methods, and this is used in the following piece of code:

```
> par(mar=c(3,3,1,1), mgp=c(3,1,0)/1.6, las=1 )
> with( plw, plot(Hurley ~ Nadler, pch=16, xlim=c(55,130), ylim=c(55,130) ) )
> abline(0,1)
> a   <- plvol.BA$reg.res["Hurley | Nadler",1]
> b   <- plvol.BA$reg.res["Hurley | Nadler",2]
> pr <- plvol.BA$reg.res["Hurley | Nadler",3]
> abline( a   , b, lwd=2, col="blue" )
> abline( a+pr, b, lwd=2, col="blue" )
> abline( a-pr, b, lwd=2, col="blue" )
> box()
```

Finally, we accommodate the fact that the standard deviation seems to increase with the mean. We regress the differences on the averages, extract the residuals and then regress the absolute values of these.

```
> m0 <- with( plw, lm( Hurley-Nadler ~ I((Hurley+Nadler)/2) ) )
> mr <- with( plw, lm( abs(residuals(m0)) ~ I((Hurley+Nadler)/2) ) )
> summary( mr )$coef
```

	Estimate	Std. Error	t value	Pr(>|t|)
(Intercept)	0.005116508	0.846141162	0.006046873	0.99518774
I((Hurley + Nadler)/2)	0.016476801	0.008909388	1.849375300	0.06744876

If we multiply the coefficients by $\sqrt{\pi/2}$ we can use them as coefficients in the linear relation of the standard deviation to the average, and we get the limits shown in Figure 4.8, which clearly does a much better job than the other attempts.

```
> sd.coef <- coef( mr ) * sqrt(pi/2)
> a.di <- plvol.BA$reg.res[1,1]
> b.di <- plvol.BA$reg.res[1,2]
> a.sd <- sd.coef[1]
> b.sd <- sd.coef[2]
> par(mar=c(3,3,1,1), mgp=c(3,1,0)/1.6, las=1 )
> with( plw, plot(Hurley ~ Nadler, pch=16, xlim=c(55,130), ylim=c(55,130)) )
> abline(0,1)
> a <- a.di
> b <- b.di
> abline( a/(1-b/2), (1+b/2)/(1-b/2), lwd=2, col="blue" )
> a <- a.di + 2*a.sd
> b <- b.di + 2*b.sd
> abline( a/(1-b/2), (1+b/2)/(1-b/2), lwd=2, col="blue" )
> a <- a.di - 2*a.sd
> b <- b.di - 2*b.sd
> abline( a/(1-b/2), (1+b/2)/(1-b/2), lwd=2, col="blue" )
> box()
```

Regression of the absolute residuals on the averages gives a non-significant slope ($P = 0.067$), but with a positive regression coefficient, indicating that standard deviations are increasing with the average. Figure 4.8 shows the prediction limits between the two methods obtained for this data set using formula (4.11). It appears that they give a more realistic set of prediction limits than do the limits based on the assumption of constant variance.

The conclusion is that explicit modeling of the standard deviation is not possible even if a simple and easily interpretable reporting of results is desired. Moreover, as we shall see in Chapter 7, the approach used here is not generalizable to the instance where replicate measurements by each method are available, and the variance can be separated into different components.

The problems with heteroscedastic errors are therefore preferably remedied by transformation of measurements.

4.8   Transformations

If the relationship between measurement methods is non-linear or if the standard deviations are not constant over the range of measurements, linearity and constant standard deviation can sometimes be obtained by transformation of the data. In some cases, constant difference between methods may come as a by-product of the transformation too.

4.8.1   Log transformation

Traditionally, the log transformation has been the first choice, because it lends itself to a reasonable interpretation of the results; differences are log ratios and averages are log-geometric means, so a Bland–Altman plot using log-transformed data can immediately be labeled in terms that relate to the original scale (see Figure 4.9).

Moreover, if the data are log-transformed, the relative scaling between methods is irrelevant since the differences between logs represent the log of the *ratio* of the two measurements. Hence the

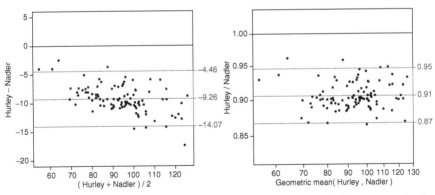

Figure 4.9   Measurements of plasma volume by two different methods. The left-hand panel has measurements on the original scale, and in the right-hand panel the measurements are log-transformed. Note how the log transformation is exploited to give interpretable labeling of the axes.

scaling problem that conceptually invalidates the regression of the differences on the averages is non-existent in this case.

It has often been argued that the log transformation is the only really usable transformation for measurement comparison data, because it is the only transform where differences on the transformed scale have meaning on the original scale, namely as ratios of measurements on the original scale – this is exploited in the labeling of the graph in the right-hand panel in Figure 4.9.

However, this point of view is based on the notion that the limits of agreement (and the Bland–Altman plot) are the only product of the method comparison. But if the plot is rotated 45° we have a plot with prediction limits for converting between the log measurements. But this plot is easily transformed back to the original scale, leaving the conversions and the prediction limits intact, albeit now not linear, but on the original scale, as shown in Figure 4.10.

Note that there is nothing special about the log transformation in this procedure; any (monotone) transformation of the data will lend

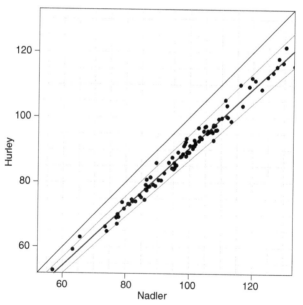

Figure 4.10 Measurements of plasma volume by two different methods. Limits of agreement for log-transformed values transformed back to the original scale – the prediction limits are applicable both ways.

itself to this procedure. What is needed is a data transformation where the conversion between methods is linear with constant variance.

Transformation of data is treated in more detail and in a more general context in Chapter 8.

4.9 Summary

If two methods are compared, and only one measurement by each is available, proceed as follows:

1. Draw a Bland–Altman plot to see if the basic assumptions for limits of agreement are met.

2. Compute limits of agreement if the basic assumptions are met. If relevant, convert to a prediction interval for one method given the other.

3. Non-constant difference between methods is detected by regressing differences on averages and checking whether the slope is 0. If there is non-constant difference, regress the differences on the means, and use the results to derive a prediction interval for one method given the other, using formulae (4.6).

4. Non-constant variance is checked by regressing the absolute residuals on the averages, and checking whether the slope is 0. If the variance is non-constant:

   • Find (preferably) a suitable transformation to resolve the problem. Create prediction intervals for one method given another and back-transform to the original scale (see details in Chapter 8).

   • Estimate the relationship of the standard deviation to the average by multiplying the coefficients from the regression of the absolute residuals on the averages by $\sqrt{\pi/2}$, and use the prediction formulae (4.11)

In any case it will be useful to also present the result as a plot for conversion between the two methods.

5

Replicate measurements

When comparing different methods of measurement, the only way to address the question of which method is better is to make sure that replicate measurements for each combination of method and item are available. Of course this cannot give a final answer to the question, but at least replicate measurements make it possible to assess the repeatability of each method. If methods do not agree on average there will of course not be any way to assess which of the methods actually does give the more correct measurements.

This chapter – large parts of which are based on Carstensen *et al.* [13] – only treats the case where the difference (bias) between methods is assumed constant; non-constant bias is treated in Chapter 7.

5.1 Pairing of replicate measurements

With replicate measurements for each combination of item and method it is not immediately clear how to plot measurements on the same item by different methods – which measurement by method 1 is plotted against which by method 2? In order to plot measurements from the two methods against each other we must decide on a pairing of the replicates. Sometimes this is inherent in the very design of the study, namely if replicates are what we call 'linked'.

Comparing Clinical Measurement Methods: A Practical Guide   Bendix Carstensen
© 2010 John Wiley & Sons, Ltd

Replicate measurements come in two substantially different forms, depending on the circumstances under which they are taken: exchangeable and linked.

5.1.1 Exchangeable replicates

Replicate measurements by a method on a given item are said to be exchangeable if there is no relationship between the first, second, etc. replicate across methods. Technically speaking, the requirement is that the distribution of data is invariant under permutation of replicate numbers *within* (method, item); this property is normally called *exchangeability* of the observations within (method, item). This will typically be the case if the replicate measurements are made independently between methods.

An example of this is the measurements of subcutaneous fat mentioned in Section 2.2.1. These data are shown in Figure 5.1. Since we have replicate measurements by both methods (in this case, observers), we must decide which replicates to match when plotting from the two methods against each other. In the left-hand part of Figure 5.1 the replication numbers as recorded in the original file are used.

Using the replicates, we can estimate the variability for each method; the intra-item standard deviation in this case is 0.077 cm for KL and 0.072 cm for SL, so the two methods (i.e. student observers) have approximately the same precision in measuring subcutaneous fat.

A naive calculation would assert that the standard deviation of the difference between measurements was $\sqrt{0.077^2 + 0.072^2} = 0.105$ cm, but the empirical standard deviation of the differences is in fact 0.135 cm when using the pairing in the data set. Thus there are sources of variation in addition to the pure measurement error. For now the limits of agreement based on the empirical standard deviation of the differences give a reasonable summary of the data; $KL - SL : 0.045 \pm 2 \times 0.135 = (-0.225; 0.315)$ cm fat.

The students who measured subcutaneous fat did it independently of each other, sometimes interchangeably. Moreover, there is no reason to suspect that the 'true' value of the subcutaneous fat changes during the course of the experiment. These two things makes it immaterial

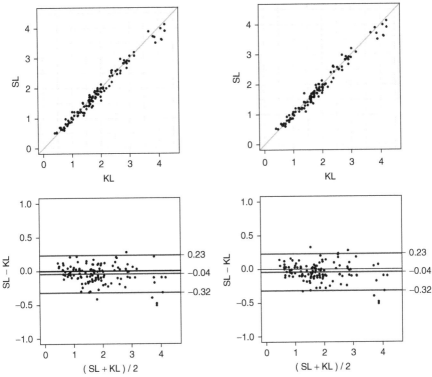

*Figure 5.1   Measurements of subcutaneous fat by two observers, KL
and SL. In the left-hand panels the replicates are matched as recorded,
in the right-hand panels a random matching of replicates has been
performed, and since replicates are indeed exchangeable no inflation
of variance is seen.*

how the replicates are numbered; the first measurement on a person
has no special status relative to the others, and replicate 1 for a given
person by KL has no special relation to any particular replicate on the
same person by SL. Thus any pairing of replicates should be as good
as any other; in fact, random pairings of replicates will in 95% of cases
give an empirical standard deviation of the differences in the interval
(0.128, 0.141) cm.

It would thus seem that a way to check whether replicates are
exchangeable is to use the definition: make a random permutation of the
replicates within (method, item) and see if the plot of the two methods
against each other looks the same. This is illustrated in Figure 5.1,

where it is clear that replicates are exchangeable, since nothing happens to the limits of agreement by permuting the replicates randomly.

However, sometimes data sets are sorted by the outcome variable, in which case the above argument breaks down; if measurements are sorted within each (method, item), the variation of differences will be artificially small, so there is no empirical basis for checking exchangeability. This is illustrated for the fat data in Figure 5.2.

Hence, there is no escape from acquiring external information on how data were collected – the information on exchangeability is not necessarily in the data set.

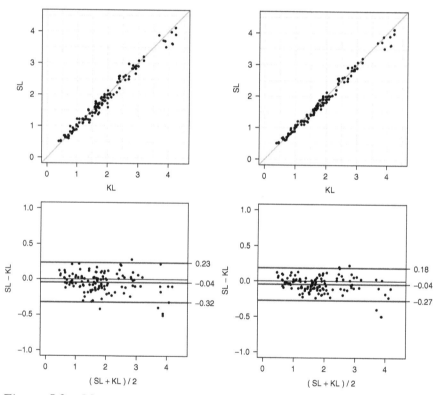

Figure 5.2   Measurements of subcutaneous fat by two observers, KL and SL. In the left-hand panels the replicates are matched as recorded, in the right-hand panels replicates have been sorted by the measured value within each (method, item), creating an artificially good agreement.

5.1.2   Linked replicates

Replicate measurements by a method on a given item are said to be linked if the first replicate measurement by one method is taken at the same time as or under some other similar special circumstances to the first replicate measurement by the other method(s). This will imply that some of the variation between replicate measurements *within* items is common for all methods. This could, for example, be the within-patient variation of blood pressure over time in a study where blood pressure is measured at certain intervals, each time by both methods.

Linked replicates may or may not be exchangeable within items (but jointly across methods). If, for example, measurement occasions represent times, there might be an effect of time such that the replicate numbers have a meaning. On the other hand, it may very well be that the link across methods is not tied to any specific feature, and so the replicate ordering is irrelevant (as long as it is the same for all methods).

At the Royal Children's Hospital in Melbourne, percentage oxygen saturation of the blood of sick children was measured by two methods: CO oximetry (involving taking a proper blood sample and analyzing it in the laboratory) and pulse oximetry (a non-invasive method using light reflection on a finger or toe). Sixty-one children were measured, most with three replicate measurements on each method, and a few with two or one. Replicates were made with some time between them, but simultaneously by the two methods.

In this case, the replicates are *linked* across methods. There are random fluctuations in the actual level of oxygen saturation, but we have no reason to expect any special development from one measuring time to the next. Therefore the *pairs* of measurements are exchangeable, but the measurements are *not* exchangeable *within* methods as in the previous example.

This is immediately visible from the two plots of the data in Figure 5.3, where we have shown data plotted with the correct linking of replicates as well as where we have randomly permuted the replicates (within each (method, item)) before plotting – the latter shows wider limits of agreement, because the variation between measuring events has erroneously been included too, even if it is irrelevant for the method comparison.

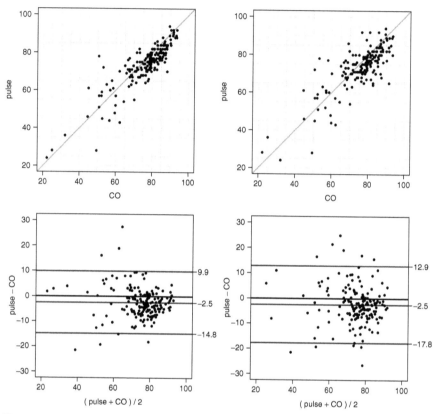

Figure 5.3   Measurements of oxygen saturation (%) in blood by CO oximetry and by pulse oximetry. In the left-hand panels the replicates are correctly matched, and in the right-hand panels a random matching of replicates has been performed, and a clear inflation of the variance is seen.

If it is known a priori that the 'true' value of the measurement will fluctuate between measurement occasions, it is desirable to choose a design where this fluctuation can be eliminated in the analysis. In the case of the oximetry measurements it would definitely have been wrong to use a design where replicates were exchangeable within methods – we would then have been unable to separate the random variation between measurement times from the residual variation ('pure' measurement error). In such a scenario we would only be able to answer questions of the type: what would the CO oximetry measurement have been for this baby *at another time point* given a pulse oximetry measurement of 83%?

5.2   Plotting replicate measurements

So far we have only plotted measurements from the two methods by pairing the replicates between methods, without indicating in the plot how the replicates belong together within items. There are two basic ways of including this information in the plot, depending on whether replicates are linked or not.

Exchangeable replicates can be shown by plotting the points $(\bar{y}_{1i\cdot}, y_{2ir})$ connected with a line, as well as $(y_{1ir}, \bar{y}_{2i\cdot})$ connected with a line. These will form a cross, and the size of the crosses in the axis directions will give an impression of the variability of replicates in the two directions. This type of plot will have one point per measurement in the data set.

Linked replicates can be shown by plotting the linked pairs of points and connecting all points (y_{1ir}, y_{2ir}), $r = 1, \ldots, R_{1i}$, by line segments to the points $(\bar{y}_{1i\cdot}, \bar{y}_{2i\cdot})$. This type of plot will have one point per *pair* of measurements in the data set.

These approaches are illustrated in Figure 5.4, including the enhancement where observations on each item are given a separate color (please see color plate section).

5.3   Models for replicate measurements

When replicate measurements are available, the aim of the analysis is exactly the same as without replicates; derivation of a prediction interval for one method given the other, or, equivalently, derivation of a prediction interval for the difference (given the average).

5.3.1   Exchangeable replicates

To derive prediction limits for differences between single measurements, we use an extension of model (4.1) for data where replicate

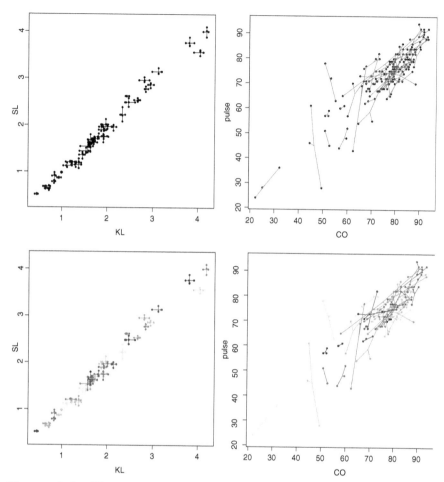

Figure 5.4 Plots of replicate measurements on each item and method. (Left) Fat data – exchangeable replicates. (Right) Oximetry data – linked replicates.

measurements are explicitly modeled:

$$y_{mir} = \alpha_m + \mu_i + c_{mi} + e_{mir}, \qquad c_{mi} \sim \mathcal{N}(0, \tau_m^2),$$

$$e_{mir} \sim \mathcal{N}(0, \sigma_m^2). \tag{5.1}$$

This is a model for *exchangeable* replicates, because there are no common terms for each combination of (item, replicate), hence the model is invariant under permutation of replicates within (method, item).

In this model we have introduced a method×item interaction, to account for possible method-specific effects of item characteristics unrelated to the actual measurements. This is the effect which we failed to take into account for the fat data when computing the within-item variation of replicates and using these to construct limits of agreement (p. 50).

In this model the variation between items for method m is modeled by the random effects c_{mi} with standard deviation τ_m and the within-item variation by σ_m. The formulation of this model is general and refers to comparison of any number of methods – however, if only two methods are compared, separate values of τ_1 and τ_2 cannot be estimated, so in the case of only two methods we are forced to assume that $\tau_1 = \tau_2 = \tau$. Another way of putting this is that we can only estimate the mean of τ_1^2 and τ_2^2, but we only ever use the sum of the variances, so the term that will be needed is $\sqrt{2\tau^2}$.

Under this model the limits of agreement should be computed based on the standard deviation of the difference between a pair of measurements by the two methods on a new item, 0, say:

$$\mathrm{var}(y_{10} - y_{20}) = \tau_1^2 + \tau_2^2 + \sigma_1^2 + \sigma_2^2.$$

Hence, the limits of agreement are estimated by

$$\hat{\alpha}_1 - \hat{\alpha}_2 \pm 2 \times \sqrt{2\hat{\tau}^2 + \hat{\sigma}_1^2 + \hat{\sigma}_2^2}.$$

Therefore it only remains to estimate the variance components in this linear mixed model and plug in the estimates in this formula.

Model (5.1) is a standard linear mixed model, and it can be fitted in most major statistical packages. For the fat data, the limits of agreement based on the parameters from the mixed model are the same to two significant digits as those derived from the pairing of measurements indicated by the numbering in the data set. We shall return to this point below.

5.3.2   Linked replicates

In the example above, we have assumed that the replicates were exchangeable *within* each method×item stratum. When replicates are taken in parallel by each of the methods, the values are linked by a common environment, typically time or sampling occasion. An example of this is the oximetry study mentioned above.

Since replicates are linked across methods, we need to incorporate this in the model by including an extra (random) effect common within each item×replicate stratum:

$$y_{mir} = \alpha_m + \mu_i + a_{ir} + c_{mi} + e_{mir},$$

$$a_{ir} \sim \mathcal{N}(0, \omega^2), \quad c_{mi} \sim \mathcal{N}(0, \tau_m^2), \quad e_{mir} \sim \mathcal{N}(0, \sigma_m^2).$$

(5.2)

Again, with only two methods we cannot estimate method-specific values for the method×item effect (τ). Also note that the variance of the extra random effect (a_{ir}) cannot depend on method; it is an extension of μ_i, and in this model the 'true' value for item i is $\mu_i + a_{ir}$.

The variance of a_{ir} represents the variation between replication conditions (common for all methods), within items. In some designs, a part of this variation may be taken out as a systematic effect (common for all items). This could, for example, be a common effect of day of analysis or the like.

When subtracting measurements by the two methods from each other, the effects a_{ir} cancel, so under this extended model the expression for the variance of the difference between a new set of measurements (on item 0, say) is

$$\mathrm{var}(y_{10} - y_{20}) = \tau_1^2 + \tau_2^2 + \sigma_1^2 + \sigma_2^2,$$

so that the limits of agreement are again estimated by

$$\hat{\alpha}_1 - \hat{\alpha}_2 \pm 2 \times \sqrt{2\hat{\tau}^2 + \hat{\sigma}_1^2 + \hat{\sigma}_2^2}.$$

(Recall that that τ^2 is the common estimate for τ_1^2 and τ_2^2.) Thus in order to produce limits of agreement we need estimates of $\alpha_1 - \alpha_2$, τ, σ_1 and σ_2.

Fixed item × replicate effect

In some cases one would introduce a fixed effect of replicate or other part of the item × replicate effect. The extreme case would be to take the effect as fixed, i.e. replace model (5.2) with

$$y_{mir} = \alpha_m + \mu_{ir} + c_{mi} + e_{mir},$$
$$c_{mi} \sim \mathcal{N}(0, \tau_m^2), \quad e_{mir} \sim \mathcal{N}(0, \sigma_m^2).$$

(5.3)

The only difference between this and a model where item × replicate is regarded as new items is the partitioning of the variance in the variation between items (τ) and the variation within items (σ). Seen in this way, it is a model for observations without replicates, and hence we cannot identify separate variances for the two methods.

Heuristically speaking, the terms $\mu_i + a_{ir}$ in model (5.2) play the role of the terms μ_{ir} in the model (5.3). The former model has the restriction that the random terms have the same variance throughout the data, so that items where the variation between replication conditions is large will have estimates of $\mu_i + a_{ir}$ (i.e. best linear unbiased predictions) that are shrunk more toward the item mean, leaving room for estimation of different residual error terms for the two methods. In a model with fixed effects of item × replicate the fitted value (μ_{ir}) is the mean of the observations by the different methods, so the residual error terms are numerically the same if only two methods are compared, and different residual variances cannot be estimated.

5.4   Interpretation of the random effects

Model (5.2) has fixed effects of item and method and two of the three two-way interactions specified as random. The method × replicate interaction is of no real interest, in particular not as a random effect. Hence, there are only the random terms method × item, item × replicate and the residual variation (the three-way interaction) as variance components to consider.

method×item: In clinical chemistry this is often called a 'matrix' effect. This refers to the soluble ('matrix') used by a specific method in the laboratory, which may interact differently with each item. The effect measures the random interactions between methods and items that may influence the outcome.

If more than two methods are compared, it will be logical to assume that the variance of this random effect depends on method, as methods may be influenced differently by matrix effects. It will only be possible to estimate separate variances for the method? item effects if more than two methods are compared.

It should be noted that the size of this variance component may depend on the choice of the items used in the experiment; a different population of items may exhibit different interactions with the methods compared.

In principle it is possible to specify a model where this effect is absent, but with replicate measurements in an experiment it is hard to see why one would lump this variance component together with the residual.

item×replicate: This effect must be included in the model if replicates are linked across methods, e.g. if replicates are taken by all methods in parallel. An example of this would be measurements by different methods, where replicates on the same persons are done on different days, say, but with all methods used each day. The item by replicate measurement would then model the random day-to-day variation within items, and induce a correlation between measurement by different methods taken on the same day.

It is necessary to include this effect in the model when replicates are linked, to accommodate the variation between replicates (within item) that is common to all methods, but the effect is in principle alien to the method comparison. We want to know how methods relate to each other if measurements are taken at the same time under similar conditions; sources of variation that do not influence the relationship *between* the methods should be kept out of the method comparisons.

method×item×replicate: The residual variation represents the pure measurement error, which is naturally expected to have method-specific variance. This is the variance component that is of primary interest when comparing methods, as it is the only one that can be said to be unrelated to the experimental design.

In the absence of replicate measurements it is impossible to separate variances of the method×item random effects from the residual errors (both are classified by method×item). Moreover, if only two methods are compared the residual (i.e. the residual *plus* the method×item) effect cannot be estimated with different variance for each method.

If replicate measurements are available, it is possible to estimate a separate residual variance for each method.

5.5   Estimation

Model (5.2) differs from model (5.1) in the *estimation* of the variance components; the formula for the prediction intervals for the differences is the same. The model where the replicates are linked across methods has some of the variation allocated to the item×replicate method – the part of the variation which is irrelevant for the method comparison.

Both (5.2) and (5.1) are standard linear mixed models (variance component models), that can be fitted in most modern software packages. The only slightly non-standard (meaning "not often used") feature is the differing residual variances between methods. It should be noted that the model with random effects of both method×item and item×replicate is a so-called "crossed" model and therefore usually will take a longer time to fit.

Chapter 12 gives code and sample output from fitting these models using some of the common software packages.

5.6   Getting it wrong and getting it almost right

If we want to directly apply the method of Bland and Altman [6] that covers the situation with only one measurement per method and item, this can be done for a data set with replicate measurements in two different ways:

1. Take means over replicates within each method×item.
2. Take replicates within item as new items.

Recall model (5.2):

$$y_{mir} = \alpha_m + \mu_i + a_{ir} + c_{mi} + e_{mir},$$

$$a_{ir} \sim \mathcal{N}(0, \omega^2), \quad c_{mi} \sim \mathcal{N}(0, \tau_m^2), \quad e_{mir} \sim \mathcal{N}(0, \sigma_m^2).$$

The random $i \times r$ interaction term is only relevant if the replicates are linked across methods (paired replicates). In the model the correct limits of agreement are

$$\alpha_1 - \alpha_2 \pm 2\sqrt{\tau_1^2 + \tau_2^2 + \sigma_1^2 + \sigma_2^2}.$$

In the case of exchangeable replicates the (item, replicate) random effect would not be in the model, but the expression for the limits of agreement would still be the same.

5.6.1 Averaging over replicates

If we are using means of replicates to form the differences, we have

$$\bar{d}_i = \bar{y}_{1i.} - \bar{y}_{2i.} = \alpha_1 - \alpha_2 + \frac{\sum_r a_{ir}}{R_{1i}} - \frac{\sum_r a_{ir}}{R_{2i}} + c_{1i} - c_{2i}$$

$$+ \frac{\sum_r e_{1ir}}{R_{1i}} - \frac{\sum_r e_{2ir}}{R_{2i}},$$

where R_{mi} is the number of replicates by method m on item i. The terms with a_{ir} are only relevant for linked replicates, in which case $R_{1i} = R_{2i}$ and therefore the term vanishes. Thus

$$\text{var}(\bar{d}_i) = \tau_1^2 + \tau_2^2 + \sigma_1^2/R_{1i} + \sigma_2^2/R_{2i} < \tau_1^2 + \tau_2^2 + \sigma_1^2 + \sigma_2^2,$$

so the limits of agreement calculated based on the means are too narrow as prediction limits for differences between future *single* measurements. Moreover, if the number of replicates is not the same for all methods and items, we cannot easily estimate this variance.

5.6.2   Replicates as items

Linked replicates

When replicates are linked we could redefine item as the cross-classification of item and replicate, in which case the calculated differences becomes

$$d_{ir} = y_{1ir} - y_{2ir} = \alpha_1 - \alpha_2 + c_{1i} - c_{2i} + e_{1ir} - e_{2ir}.$$

These differences have variances $\tau_1^2 + \tau_2^2 + \sigma_1^2 + \sigma_2^2$, and therefore using the empirical variance of the differences apparently gives the correct limits of agreement. However, the differences are not independent (as would have been the case if replicates were from different items):

$$\mathrm{cov}(d_{ir}, d_{is}) = \tau_1^2 + \tau_2^2, \qquad \mathrm{corr}(d_{ir}, d_{is}) = \frac{\tau_1^2 + \tau_2^2}{\tau_1^2 + \tau_2^2 + \sigma_1^2 + \sigma_2^2}.$$

This is negligible if the residual variances are very large compared to the interaction. But this is not necessarily the case so the estimate of the 'correct' variance based on these differences is likely to be biased downward. The downward bias is because the empirical variance of a sample with positive intercorrelation is smaller than that of a sample (with the same marginal variance) and zero intercorrelation.

Exchangeable replicates

If replicates are exchangeable within method×item it is not clear how to produce the differences – it can be done in a number of different ways since the replicates can be matched within item in several different ways. If replicates are paired at random, the variance will still be correct, assuming model (5.1),

$$\mathrm{var}(y_{1ir} - y_{2is}) = \tau_1^2 + \sigma_1^2 + \tau_2^2 + \sigma_2^2,$$

but again the differences will be positively correlated within item,

$$\mathrm{cov}(y_{1ir} - y_{2is}, y_{1it} - y_{2iu}) = \tau_1^2 + \tau_2^2,$$

so the estimate of $\tau_1^2 + \sigma_1^2 + \tau_2^2 + \sigma_2^2$ as the empirical variance of $y_{1ir} - y_{2is}$ for a random matching of replicates between methods will be an underestimate, albeit not a large one. In the fat data set (with exchangeable replicates) the correct upper limit of agreement based on the model is 0.315, the upper limit based on pairing induced by the numbering in the data set is 0.312, but the median upper limit over 1000 random matchings of replicates within items is 0.309.

5.7 Summary

If two methods of measurement are compared, and replicate measurements are available for each combination of method and item, proceed as follows:

1. Establish whether replicates are linked. This cannot be determined based on the data alone; it is a function of the study design.

2. If replicates are:

   - exchangeable, make a random pairing of the replicates across methods;

   - linked, use the pairing of replicates given in the design.

3. Draw a Bland–Altman plot using the item×replicate as plotting unit (i.e. as items).

4. Check for non-constant difference between methods by regressing the differences on the average. If the differences are not constant refer to the methods in Chapter 7.

5. Check for non-constant variance by regressing the absolute values of the residuals (from the previous regression) on the averages. If the variance is non-constant, find a suitable transformation of the measurements that makes the variance of the differences constant.

6. If the differences and the variances are constant, fit the appropriate variance component model to (the transformed) data with random effects of method×item and if replicates are linked also item×replicate. Use estimates to construct limits of agreement.

6

Several methods of measurement

Sometimes more than two methods are compared. The initial approach would be to make pairwise comparisons of methods, but it would of course be more satisfactory to make a comparison of all methods in one model, to ensure that the estimated difference between method 1 and 3 was equal to the sum of the difference between methods 1 and 2 and the difference between methods 2 and 3.

Before this is done, however, consideration should be given to whether some of the methods are more similar than others. In the extreme case, we may have two methods which produce very similar results but are highly inaccurate. If these are compared to a third accurate method it may happen that the accurate method is deemed inaccurate in comparison with the other two.

6.1 Model

The model we set up for method comparisons (5.2) with replicate measurements is generalizable to several methods of measurement:

$$y_{mir} = \alpha_m + \mu_i + a_{ir} + c_{mi} + e_{mir},$$
$$a_{ir} \sim \mathcal{N}(0, \omega^2), \quad c_{mi} \sim \mathcal{N}(0, \tau_m^2), \quad e_{mir} \sim \mathcal{N}(0, \sigma_m^2).$$

Comparing Clinical Measurement Methods: A Practical Guide Bendix Carstensen
© 2010 John Wiley & Sons, Ltd

The model merely states that there is a constant difference between methods, and they have separate measurement errors (σ_m^2). Moreover, it is assumed that the method×item (matrix) effects have different variances between methods as well. Depending on the context this may or may not be a feasible assumption, and use of a model may be considered where $\text{var}(c_{mi}) = \tau^2$, independent of method.

Limits of agreement between any two methods (2 and 1, say) are computed as in the case of two methods only,

$$\alpha_2 - \alpha_1 \pm 2 \times \sqrt{\tau_1^2 + \tau_2^2 + \sigma_1^2 + \sigma_2^2};$$

and, by the same token, prediction of measurement by method 2 given a measurement by method 1 is (with a 95% prediction interval)

$$y_{2|1} = y_1 + \alpha_2 - \alpha_1 \pm 2 \times \sqrt{\tau_1^2 + \tau_2^2 + \sigma_1^2 + \sigma_2^2}.$$

The joint model for three or more methods gives the same mean differences between pairs of methods as we would get by using only the data from each pair of methods; they are merely the differences of the means of each method, except for special (uncommon) cases where some items lack measurements on one method.

6.2   Replicate measurements

In the case of replicate measurements, it is possible to separate the residual variation and the method×item variation, and, if more than two methods are compared, to allow the latter to have method-specific variance too. It is of course still necessary to estimate an item×replicate variance if replicates are linked across methods.

The introduction of a third method allows the separation of the method×item variation between the methods. In the case of only two methods the deviations of the empirical method means for a given item can only be taken to be of opposite sign from the method×item means $\mu_i + \alpha_m$ (this is how μ_i is determined). But with three methods, we have three different distances to the method×item means. So this separation of the method×item variation by method is crucially dependent on the assumption that the methods measure the same quantity, and that the measurements by different methods are independent (given the "true" values of course).

As mentioned above, the effect of having two methods that are strongly correlated compared with a third one may be that the third one is deemed inaccurate even if the two correlated methods are *in*accurate. There is no way to detect this phenomenon from an observed body of data; the data would look exactly the same if two independent accurate methods were compared to a third inaccurate method.

6.3   Single measurement by each method

Even if there is only a single measurement by each method it is actually possible to fit a model with a constant difference between methods and separate residual variances if more than two methods are compared. In the absence of replicates the residual variation e_{mi} and the matrix effects c_{mi} cannot be separated – they both appear as part of the residual interaction, so only the parameters $\sqrt{\tau_m^2 + \sigma_m^2}$ can be identified. The effect of linked replicates (a_{ir}) will in the absence of replicates of course be irrelevant.

Hence the only effect of comparing more than two methods with only a single measurement on each is that it is possible to estimate the sum of the matrix variance and the residual variance for each method separately. This possibility is, however, heavily dependent on the assumption that the methods are measuring the same quantity, and that the matrix effects are independent between methods.

If matrix effects for two out of three methods are very correlated, an analysis ignoring this will produce small variances for these two methods and a larger variance for the third method, because a part if the matrix effect is absorbed in the fixed effect of item. But there is no way to reveal such effects using recorded data alone if variances are allowed to depend on method.

7

A general model for method comparisons

In this section we first discuss the model and its use as if estimates of the parameters were available. Subsequently, estimation procedures are discussed.

In some method comparison studies, the difference between methods will vary with the measurement level. The simplest way to accommodate such variation is to allow a linear relationship between measurements. This is done in the following general model where we assume that measurements by each method depend linearly on the 'true' value for the item, μ_i:

$$y_{mir} = \alpha_m + \beta_m \left(\mu_i + a_{ir} + c_{mi} \right) + e_{mir},$$
$$a_{ir} \sim \mathcal{N}(0, \omega^2), \quad c_{mi} \sim \mathcal{N}(0, \tau_m^2), \quad e_{mir} \sim \mathcal{N}(0, \sigma_m^2) \tag{7.1}$$

with $m = 1, \ldots, M$, $i = 1, \ldots, I$, and $r = 1, \ldots, R_{mi}$.

Data can be viewed as organized in a three-way layout, classified by method, item and replicate. The model has main effects of method (α_m), item (μ_i) and a fixed interaction between method and item ($\beta_m \mu_i$), the latter is only a *part* of the full interaction, so there is still room for a random method×item interaction (c_{mi}) accounting for the rest. As for the models with constant bias, an item×replicate effect is included to

Comparing Clinical Measurement Methods: A Practical Guide   Bendix Carstensen
© 2010 John Wiley & Sons, Ltd

accommodate linked replicates. There is no fixed effect of replicate, although this may easily be incorporated. Only two of the three two-way interactions are included as random effects; the method×item effect (c_{mi}) and the item×replicate effect (a_{ir}).

Model (7.1) is an extension of model (5.2) on page 50, where the additive mean $\alpha_m + \mu_i$ is replaced by $\alpha_m + \beta_m\mu_i$, as in model (4.2) on page 24. This makes the extended model non-linear in the fixed parameters, and also introduces terms where fixed parameters are multiplied by the random effects ($\beta_m a_{ir}$ and $\beta_m c_{mi}$).

The parameter μ_i can be thought of as the underlying (but unobserved) true measurement value for item i, and α_m and β_m are the parameters that define the linear relationship between μ_i and the mean of the measurement on item i made by method m, and hence also between the methods of measurement. The model as formulated in (7.1) is overparametrized, but we shall return to the implications of this below.

7.1   Scaling

Model (7.1) is qualitatively different from the two-way analysis of variance model (4.1) or the more elaborate model with all variance components (5.2) where $\beta_m = 1$ for all m, where there is a fixed *constant difference* between measurements by different methods. When the β_ms are allowed to vary freely as in (7.1), the methods are *scaled* relative to each other.

Models (4.1), (5.1) and (5.2) assume that all methods measure on the same scale. This is why differences between measurements by different methods are meaningful. But introducing the relative scaling of methods as in (7.1) makes differences between measurements by different methods meaningless. Model (7.1) is invariant under rescaling of measurements from one method; if, for example, the y_1s were all multiplied by 2, then we would just get α_1, β_1 and σ_1 twice as big, the other parameters in the model would be the same and the relationship between methods would be the same. Thus under model (7.1) it is in principle only meaningful to form differences between methods after rescaling to the same units, i.e. by dividing measurements by β_m.

7.2   Interpretation of the random effects

The general model (7.1) has at first glance the same random effects as model (5.2) with constant difference between methods, but because of the scaling between methods introduced by the βs a little more care is needed in the interpretation of the random effects.

method×item: The model is formulated with a scaling of this random effect by the βs. This is necessary if we want to allow for a version of the model where the matrix effect is identical across methods, which is necessary in the case of two methods, and occasionally desirable for $M > 2$. Therefore this effect should be reported on an interpretable scale, i.e. as a random effect with standard deviation $\beta_m \tau$ or $\beta_m \tau_m$, depending on the choice of model.

   If the random effects c_{mi} were not scaled by the βs, the model would not be invariant under rescaling of the measurements from one method if the variance was constant across methods, and therefore would not be meaningful for comparison of methods. A major flaw in the paper by Carstensen [10] is that this aspect has been overlooked, so the models discussed there are formally meaningless.

item×replicate: This random effect can be interpreted as the random variation of the true values between replication instances. Thus it is necessary to model any systematic variation between replications explicitly if it is part of the design.

   Since the general linear structure of the relationship between methods formally allows methods to measure on different scales, this random effect (common for all methods) must also necessarily be on the 'dimensionless' scale of the μs.

   Since the μs, the αs and the βs are only determined up to a linear/scale transformation (see Section 7.3), the size of the variance component ω is not meaningful in itself. It is only interpretable when scaled to a particular method as $\beta_m \omega$.

method×item×replicate: The residual error poses no particular problems as it will always be assumed to have a standard deviation that depends on measurement method.

7.3   Parametrization of the mean

The linear relationship linking the methods in model (7.1) gives the following (mean) translation formula between two methods (1 and 2, say):

$$y_2 = \alpha_2 + \beta_2 \mu = \alpha_2 + \beta_2(y_1 - \alpha_1)/\beta_1 = \left(\alpha_2 - \alpha_1\frac{\beta_2}{\beta_1}\right) + \frac{\beta_2}{\beta_1}y_1$$

i.e. the intercept and slope used for conversion from method 1 to 2 are

$$y_2 = \alpha_{2|1} + \beta_{2|1}y_1,$$

where

$$\alpha_{2|1} = \alpha_2 - \alpha_1\frac{\beta_2}{\beta_1}, \qquad \beta_{2|1} = \frac{\beta_2}{\beta_1}.$$

These are the functions of the model parameters that are of interest – the parameters in model (7.1) are merely tools reflecting our opinion on how data were generated.

As mentioned above, model (7.1) is overparametrized – a linear transformation of the μs will just result in a linear transformation of the αs and βs; a transformation $\mu_i \mapsto \xi_i = \gamma + \delta\mu_i$ leads to the formulation

$$y_{mi} = \alpha_m + \beta_m\mu_i = \alpha_m + \beta_m(\xi_i - \gamma)/\delta = (\alpha_m - \beta_m\gamma/\delta) + (\beta_m/\delta)\xi_i$$
$$= \tilde{\alpha}_m + \tilde{\beta}_m\xi_i.$$

However, $\alpha_{2|1}$ and $\beta_{2|1}$ are invariant under replacement of α_m by $\tilde{\alpha}_m$ and β_m by $\tilde{\beta}_m$:

$$\tilde{\alpha}_{2|1} = \tilde{\alpha}_2 - \tilde{\alpha}_1\frac{\tilde{\beta}_2}{\tilde{\beta}_1}$$
$$= (\alpha_2 - \beta_2\gamma/\delta) - (\alpha_1 - \beta_1\gamma/\delta)(\beta_2/\delta)/(\beta_1/\delta)$$
$$= (\alpha_2 - \beta_2\gamma/\delta) - \left(\alpha_1\frac{\beta_2}{\beta_1} - \beta_2\gamma/\delta\right)$$
$$= \alpha_2 - \alpha_1\frac{\beta_2}{\beta_1} = \alpha_{2|1},$$

$$\tilde{\beta}_{2|1} = \frac{\tilde{\beta}_2}{\tilde{\beta}_1}$$

$$= \frac{\beta_2/\delta}{\beta_1/\delta}$$

$$= \frac{\beta_2}{\beta_1} = \beta_{2|1}.$$

The overparametrization of the model is thus irrelevant for the conversion equations between the methods – any reparametrization will produce the same conversion equation between methods; the values $\alpha_{2|1}$ and $\beta_{2|1}$ will be the same. It has the advantage that the formulation of the model is symmetric in methods, but the drawback is that it is not directly useful for implementation in standard statistical software.

Moreover, if all measurements by one method are rescaled (e.g. converted from mmol/l to mg/dl as is common in blood glucose measurement), the conversion equations will reflect this.

7.4   Prediction limits

Model (7.1) provides a linear conversion between method means, but also a way to compute prediction limits between methods; recall the model formulation

$$y_{mir} = \alpha_m + \beta_m (\mu_i + a_{ir} + c_{mi}) + e_{mir}.$$

For a potential measurement on a new item, 0, say, by method 2, y_{20} (omitting replicate number) is given by

$$y_{20} = \alpha_2 + \beta_2(\mu_0 + a_0 + c_{20}) + e_{20}.$$

A measurement by method 1, y_{10}, is under the model assumed related to the 'true' value by

$$y_{10} = \alpha_1 + \beta_1(\mu_0 + a_0 + c_{10}) + e_{10} \quad \Rightarrow$$

$$\mu_0 = \frac{y_{10} - \alpha_1 - \beta_1 c_{10} - e_{10}}{\beta_1} - a_0.$$

This is the same argument as in Section 4.1, p. 22; the observation y_{10} is the only one with information on the unknown quantity μ_0 and hence the prediction

$$y_{20} = \alpha_2 + \beta_2(\mu_0 + a_0 + c_{20}) + e_{20}$$

$$= \alpha_2 + \beta_2 \left(\frac{y_{10} - \alpha_1 - \beta_1 c_{10} - e_{10}}{\beta_1} - a_0 + a_0 + c_{20} \right) + e_{20}$$

$$= \left(\alpha_2 - \alpha_1 \frac{\beta_2}{\beta_1} \right) + \frac{\beta_2}{\beta_1} y_{10} - \frac{\beta_2}{\beta_1}(\beta_1 c_{10} - e_{10}) + \beta_2 c_{20} + e_{20}$$

$$= \alpha_{2|1} + \beta_{2|1} y_{01} - \beta_2/\beta_1(\beta_1 c_{10} + e_{10}) + \beta_2 c_{20} + e_{20}.$$

Note that the random individual$\times$replicate term $a_{ir} = a_0$ vanishes from these calculations. This is because the new (single) observation is assumed to come from the same item and same replicate and thus the (item, replicate) specific terms cancel out by subtraction.

Finally, by taking the variance of the right-hand side of the equation and ignoring the estimation error in the αs and βs we have

$$\text{s.d.}(y_{2|1}) = \sqrt{(\beta_2/\beta_1)^2(\beta_1^2 \tau_1^2 + \sigma_1^2) + (\beta_2^2 \tau_2^2 + \sigma_2^2)} \qquad (7.2)$$

and, by symmetry,

$$\text{s.d.}(y_{1|2}) = \sqrt{(\beta_1^2 \tau_1^2 + \sigma_1^2) + (\beta_1/\beta_2)^2(\beta_2^2 \tau_2^2 + \sigma_2^2)} = \text{s.d.}(y_{2|1}) \times \frac{\beta_1}{\beta_2}.$$

The prediction limits for the conversion from method 1 to method 2 are therefore

$$y_{2|1} = \alpha_{2|1} + \beta_{2|1} y_1 \pm 2 \times \text{s.d.}(y_{2|1}).$$

The vertical distance between the line and the limits is $2 \times \text{s.d.}(y_{2|1})$, so the horizontal distance is obtained by division by the slope:

$$2 \times \text{s.d.}(y_{2|1})/\beta_{2|1} = 2 \times \text{s.d.}(y_{2|1})\frac{\beta_1}{\beta_2} = 2 \times \text{s.d.}(y_{1|2}).$$

Therefore a plot of the conversion line with prediction limits is applicable both ways.

The model is formulated such that it makes sense even with only two methods, where it is impossible to estimate separate variances for the matrix effects or where matrix effects are just assumed constant across methods for want of data. In this formulation, the standard deviations of the matrix effects (τs) are on the arbitrary μ-scale and hence need to be scaled to the proper measurement units by the relevant βs.

7.4.1   Mean of replicates

In the event that a prediction of a mean over K replicates by method 2 is to be predicted from an observed mean over N replicates by method 1, a slight modification is needed. The method$\times$item effects would be the same across replicates, but the error terms would differ, and the relevant prediction standard deviation would be

$$\text{s.d.}(y_{2|1}) = \sqrt{(\beta_2/\beta_1)^2(\beta_1\tau_1^2 + \sigma_1^2/N) + (\beta_2\tau_2^2 + \sigma_2^2/K)}.$$

7.4.2   Plotting predictions between methods

Once estimates of the parameters of the model have been obtained, the relationships between methods can be reported. This can either be in the form of the equations linking the means and the prediction standard deviation, or more conveniently in the form of a plot showing how measurement by one method can be predicted from those by another. Obviously, this requires a plot for every pair of methods.

In a plot of this kind, one would also insert the estimated conversion equations with prediction intervals (see Figure 7.1). Note that this graph is merely for illustration, we have not so far covered how to arrive at these estimates.

7.4.3   Reporting variance components

Model (7.1) has three variance components (the residual, method$\times$item and item$\times$replicate); but at the same time the model has observations

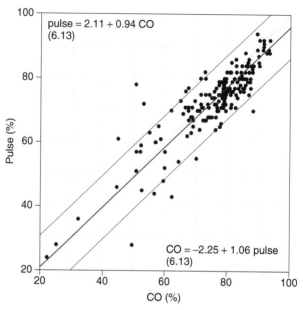

Figure 7.1   Prediction between methods of measurement of oxygen saturation in sick children. The prediction lines and 95% limits are applicable both ways. Each dot represents a pair of linked replicate measurements; each child contributes three points.

on separate scales for each method. It will therefore only make sense to report the variance components on the scales where measurements are actually taken.

The residual variances are always estimated separately for each method, as the model is formulated directly in the units of the respective measurement scales.

The matrix effects (method$\times$item) are estimated on the arbitrary scale of the μs, and hence their standard deviation must be reported as $\beta_m \tau_m$. In those cases where the variances of the matrix effects are assumed identical for all methods (on the arbitrary scale, equal to τ) we would still be reporting different variance components, $\beta_m \tau$.

The variation between replicates within items, the item$\times$replicate effect, is also on this arbitrary scale, and therefore also must be reported separately on each of the measurement scales; the ratio of the reported values will correspond to the slopes linking the methods. So in addition to the mean value parameters there is only one extra parameter for this variance component.

Hence, reporting of variance components will always be as three standard deviations on each of the scales.

7.4.4   Comparison with a gold standard

Using the general model (7.1) we have the prediction equation between two methods:

$$y_{2|1} = \alpha_{2|1} + \beta_{2|1} y_{10} \pm 2\sqrt{(\beta_2/\beta_1)^2 (\beta_1^2 \tau_1^2 + \sigma_1^2) + (\beta_2^2 \tau_2^2 + \sigma_2^2)}.$$

If we consider method 2 to be the gold standard, we may make the rather bold assumption that $\tau_2 = \sigma_2 = 0$. In this case the relationship of model (7.1) can be derived from regression of y_1 (the new, imperfect method) on y_2 (the gold standard without error), the residual standard deviation σ_{res}, say, being an estimate of $\beta_1^2 \tau_1^2 + \sigma_1^2$, and the parameters estimates of $\alpha_{1|2}$, $\beta_{1|2}$. By this token we can predict a measurement by the gold standard method (method 2) from the imperfect method (method 1) using the prediction formula (7.2):

$$y_{20} = \alpha_{2|1} + \beta_{2|1} y_{10} \pm 2\sqrt{(\beta_2/\beta_1)^2 (\beta_1^2 \tau_1^2 + \sigma_1^2)}$$
$$= \alpha_{2|1} + \beta_{2|1} y_{10} \pm 2\beta_{2|1}\sigma_{res}.$$

Thus, comparison with a gold standard where we allow for non-constant bias can be done by regressing the imperfect method on the gold standard and using the resulting regression with prediction limits to predict the other way round, i.e. the values of the gold standard from measurements by the imperfect method. This involves inverting the regression equation and adjusting the prediction standard deviation.

The assumption underlying this is that both the residual standard deviation as well as the standard deviation of the method×item interaction are 0. The former may not be too unrealistic in certain circumstances (it may well be a mere question of definition), whereas the latter seems a bit more unrealistic, although this can be considered a matter of definition too. So even if it seems at face value a sensible solution to regress the imperfect method on the gold standard, the underlying assumptions may be quite bold in many practical circumstances.

The regression approach is superfluous if replicate measurements are present, because all variance components can then be identified. But in the case where no replicate measurements are available, the general model provides a framework for understanding the assumptions made when regressing the imperfect measurement on the gold standard. Hence, traditional regression *may* be useful for something in this context, but only on the assumption (or definition) of zero method×item and zero residual variation for the gold standard.

7.5   Estimation

The general model (7.1) was defined by

$$y_{mir} = \alpha_m + \beta_m \left(\mu_i + a_{ir} + c_{mi}\right) + e_{mir}.$$

This is a variance component model with a mean which is non-linear in the parameters (because of the $\beta_m \mu_i$ term), and therefore does not easily lend itself to estimation in standard statistical software. Moreover, the model is for symmetry reasons formulated with an overparametrized mean. A constraint such as $\alpha_1 = 0$, $\beta_1 = 1$ would solve this, but it would lose the symmetry.

However, it turns out that the symmetric specification of the model allows for an ad-hoc algorithm for estimation, which bypasses the problems of overparametrization connected to estimation (but of course not the problems related to reporting).

7.5.1   Alternating regressions

This estimation method exploits the fact that estimation in model (7.1) is simple if either of two subsets of the parameters are known. Alternating between formulations makes it possible to break down the estimation into two simple steps. The ideas in this section are based on a paper by Carstensen [10], although that paper contained substantial misunderstandings.

There are two iteration steps in fitting the model, in each of which different sets of parameters are fixed and the rest estimated; hence the name 'alternating regressions'.

1. If we assume that the terms $\zeta_{mir} = \mu_i + a_{ir} + c_{mi}$ are known, then the model yields separate models for each method, each of which is a simple regression of y_{mir} on ζ_{mir}:

$$y_{mir} = \alpha_m + \beta_m \zeta_{mir} + e_{mir}, \qquad e_{mir} \sim \mathcal{N}(0, \sigma_m^2).$$

   Fitting these models will give estimates of α_m, β_m and σ_m, *conditional* on the chosen ζs. Starting values for the ζ_{mir} could conveniently be taken as the fitted values from a fixed effects model with terms $(m \times i)$ and, if needed, $(i \times r)$.

   In the estimation here we assume that the ζs are known, but the terms in ζ_{mir} actually contains $I - 2$ fixed parameters – the -2 being due to the overparametrization explained in Section 7.3. Hence the number of degrees of freedom used for estimation of the residual variance is too large, so the estimates will be biased toward 0. So the variance estimates (σ_m) from this iteration step cannot not be used without correction.

2. If, on the other hand, the estimates of the αs and βs are taken as known the model can be rearranged to the scale of the underlying μs:

$$\frac{y_{mir} - \alpha_m}{\beta_m} = \mu_i + a_{ir} + c_{mi} + e_{mir}/\beta_m,$$

$$a_{ir} \sim \mathcal{N}(0, \omega^2), \quad c_{mi} \sim \mathcal{N}(0, \tau_m^2), \quad e_{mir} \sim \mathcal{N}(0, \sigma_m^2).$$

   Taking the left-hand side as the response, we have a linear random effects model that can be used to update the estimates of the μs, and to estimate the variance components ω, τ_m and σ_m; the latter by multiplying the residual standard deviations by β_m. Finally, the best linear unbiased predictors for a_{ir} and c_{mi} can be extracted and used to update the ζs.

The model fitted in this step has I fixed parameters, but the actual number of fixed parameters in model (7.1) is $2M + I - 2$, so the variance components will have too many degrees of freedom when fitted in standard software, and hence are slightly underestimated. The fixed effects in the model, $\alpha_m + \beta_m \mu_i$, are in the method×item stratum, so the degrees of freedom for the method×item random effect are overestimated, hence the variance estimates should be adjusted accordingly (inflated a little). The following approximate variance analysis diagram for the general model illustrates this:

$$[M \times I \times R]^{MIR}_{MIR-MI-IR}$$

$$[M \times I]^{MI}_{MI-2M-I+2} \longrightarrow (\alpha_m + \beta_m \mu_i)^{2M+I-2}_{2M-2}$$

$$[I \times R]^{IR}_{IR-I} \longrightarrow (\mu_i)^I_I$$

$$(7.3)$$

In this display, the random effects are in square brackets, and the fixed effects in parentheses. The superscripts refer to the number of levels, whereas the subscripts refer to the degrees of freedom.

The estimates of the τs (the method×item standard deviations) from the algorithm have too many degrees of freedom; the extra $2M - 2$ parameters from the αs and βs are ignored; the estimates of the τs from the algorithm should therefore be adjusted by a factor $(MI - I)/(MI - 2M - I + 2) = I/(I - 2)$.

The process can then be iterated to convergence, using some measure of change of parameters as convergence criterion. The linear dependence among the parameters (α_m, β_m) and μ_i is conveniently bypassed by this estimation algorithm, since the two sets of parameters estimated in each step are fully identifiable in each of the steps. However, convergence cannot be evaluated at the scale of these indeterminate parameters because there is no guarantee that the μ_is do not wander off to infinity while the α_ms and β_ms approach 0 or vice versa. In practice the estimates of (α_m, β_m) should therefore be converted to the parameters linking the methods (which *are* identifiable), and convergence assessed using these. Likewise the variance component estimates should be converted to the actual measurement scales when evaluating convergence of the process.

Heuristic explanation

The first step of the iteration algorithm assumes that the true values $\mu_i + a_{ir} + c_{mi}$ are known, hence it is straightforward to estimate the relationship of each of the methods to this, producing estimates of α_m and β_m as well as residual variances.

In the second step the 'true values' are re-estimated in order to fit the data; the observations y_{mir} are assumed to be scattered around M lines (with known intercept α_m and slope β_m) as functions of the μ_is. The second iteration step basically moves the μ_is around to produce the best possible fit for all M lines simultaneously. It is of course always possible to reshuffle the μ_is so that the $\bar{y}_{mi}$.s from one method are perfectly on a straight line. Occasionally we may therefore see a perfect fit for one of lines, in which case corresponding estimate of the variance component $\tau_m = $ s.d.(c_{mi}) becomes 0. This means that the algorithm occasionally will produce non-credible results by letting one (or more) of the τs go to 0.

The AltReg function

This estimation method is implemented in the AltReg function in the MethComp package for R. A small simulation example based on 500 simulated data sets with 30 items and three methods with three exchangeable replicate measurements by each clearly shows that instabilities do occur in some cases.

Judging from Figure 7.2, the algorithm performs reasonably well, with the occasional instability that renders one of the variances 0.

The alternating regressions algorithm does not produce confidence intervals for the parameters. Moreover, the mean parameters of interest are non-linear functions of the parameters actually fitted, and no

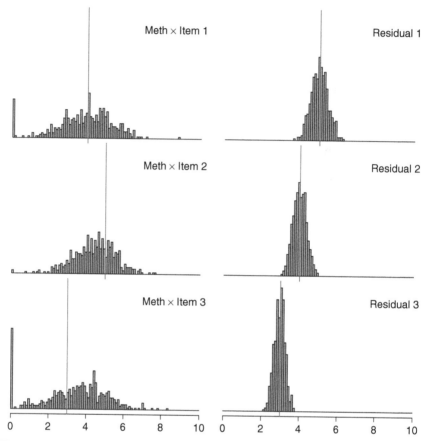

Figure 7.2   Estimates from 500 data sets simulated with the same vari-ance components. Replicates were assumed exchangeable. The red lines (please see color plate section) indicate the values of the variance components used in the simulation. The occasional instability giving method×item variance components equal to 0 is evident.

usable uncertainty of the variance components comes from the random effects models.

For a set of estimates we can of course produce a conversion algorithm with prediction intervals; this only requires estimates of the mean parameters (αs and βs) and the variance components.

But assessing the precision of the methods beyond this would require some kind of handle on the uncertainly of the variance estimates, which is not provided by the output from the alternating regressions. This could be remedied by using a bootstrap procedure, but putting a bootstrap on top of the proposed iterative procedure would be computationally quite intensive. So in this light the natural step would be to use Markov chain Monte Carlo (MCMC) methods as implemented in BUGS.

7.5.2 Estimation using BUGS

One possibility to remedy the lack of precision estimates for the variance components is to resort to bootstrapping, but given that computer-intensive methods are needed anyway, it would be natural to use the available machinery for Bayesian inference implemented in BUGS,[1] which will give posterior distributions for any desired function of the parameters of the model specified.

BUGS has the advantage that the specification of the model need not be of full rank, i.e. an overparametrized model is allowed. It is of course another matter whether such a model specification for a particular data set will produce a Markov chain that converges to the correct stationary distribution.

The problem with the overparametrized model is that the simulated chains for the μ_is may wander off to infinity while the βs get ever closer to 0 (or vice versa), eventually causing problems with precision. Likewise, the random effects would be inflated (although not the residuals). This can be fixed by choosing a prior for the μ_i with finite support, say the interval from 0 to 100. This will induce a posterior with support in the same interval and the problem will be solved.

The priors for the variance components are specified as largely uninformative, as uniform on an interval from 0 to a sufficiently large number. The αs are given flat normal priors with mean 0 and the βs a uniform prior on the interval [0, 10].

Running this model in BUGS will produce posterior samples for all the parameters in the model. These can then be used to compute

---

[1] In this context BUGS is used as a generic term for various implementations of this language and associated MCMC methods such as Classic BUGS, WinBUGS, R2WinBUGS, BRugs and JAGS.

posterior samples from the parameters of interest, $\alpha_{1|2}$, $\beta_{1|2}$, σ_1, σ_2, etc. The posterior medians of these can then be used as estimates when deriving the conversion equations between the methods.

Posterior medians for the intercept and slope

When reporting the results it would be preferable to have *one* conversion equation for each pair of methods, i.e. all conversion parameters should fulfill

$$\alpha_{1|2} = -\alpha_{2|1}/\beta_{2|1} \quad \text{and} \quad \beta_{1|2} = 1/\beta_{2|1}.$$

The latter is automatically fulfilled for the posterior medians of the slopes because

$$\frac{1}{\text{median}(\beta_{2|1})} = \text{median}\left(\frac{1}{\beta_{2|1}}\right) = \text{median}(\beta_{1|2}),$$

a simple consequence of the fact that the inverse is a monotone function and that $\beta_{2|1} = 1/\beta_{1|2}$ in all posterior samples. For other quantiles of the posterior we have similar results (allowing for the fact the inverse is a decreasing function).

But this nice property does not hold for the intercept parameters, because both αs and βs are involved; in all the posterior samples we have $\alpha_{2|1} = -\alpha_{1|2}/\beta_{1|2}$, but since this is not a simple monotone transformation we will see that

$$\text{median}(\alpha_{1|2}) \neq -\text{median}(\alpha_{2|1})/\text{median}(\beta_{2|1}).$$

In order to remedy this, a sensible compromise would therefore be to use

$$\tilde{\alpha}_{1|2} = \left(\text{median}(\alpha_{1|2}) + \text{median}(-\alpha_{2|1})/\text{median}(\beta_{2|1})\right)/2.$$

Multiplying this by $\text{median}(\beta_{2|1}) = 1/\text{median}(\beta_{1|2})$ leads to

$$\left(\text{median}(\alpha_{1|2})/\text{median}(\beta_{1|2}) + \text{median}(-\alpha_{2|1})\right)/2 = \tilde{\alpha}_{2|1}.$$

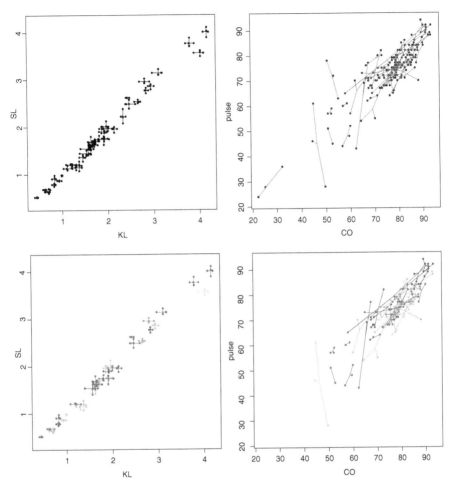

Figure 5.4   Plots of replicate measurements on each item and method. (Left) Fat data – exchangeable replicates. (Right) Oximetry data – linked replicates.

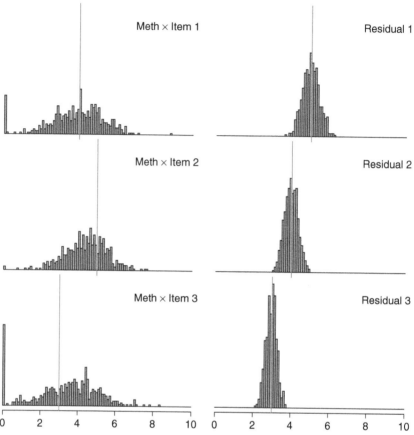

Figure 7.2   Estimates from 500 data sets simulated with the same variance components. Replicates were assumed exchangeable. The red lines indicate the values of the variance components used in the simulation. The occasional instability giving method×item variance components equal to 0 is evident.

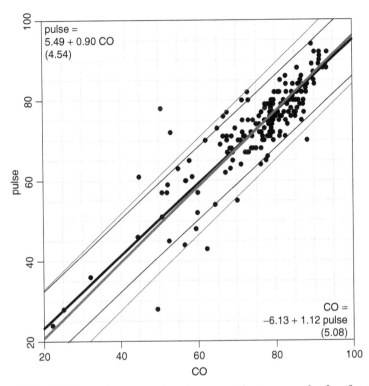

Figure 7.3   Estimated conversion between the two methods of measuring oxygen saturation. The black line and black text are based on the posterior medians from a Monte Carlo chain simulation. The blue lines are based on the estimates from the alternating regressions procedure.

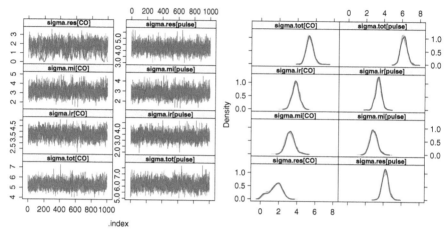

Figure 7.4   Monitoring of the posterior distributions of the estimates of the variance components from the oximetry data.

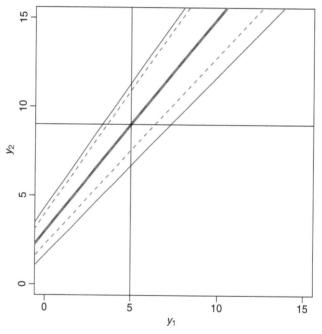

Figure 7.5   Example of prediction limits when the relationship between methods is as in equation (7.4). The blue lines refer to the prediction of y_2 from y_1 and the dotted red lines to the predictions the other way round.

Hence, the quantity computed this way gives the same intercepts regardless of whether we compute it as $\tilde{\alpha}_{1|2}$ and convert to $\tilde{\alpha}_{2|1}$ or vice versa.

The MCmcmc function

The procedure described above is implemented by the function MCmcmc in the MethComp package for R. The function takes a specification of the model as input, and then writes the necessary BUGS code and runs this using the R2WinBUGS machinery, either using WinBUGS or OpenBUGS.

7.5.3   A worked example

Oximetry data

The following shows how the tools provided in the MethComp package are used in the analysis of the oximetry data. The functions that provide estimates in the models discussed so far are BA.est, AltReg and MCmcmc.

First we load the MethComp package:

```
> library( MethComp )
```

We can then get the oximetry data (a data frame) and designate it as a Meth object, which will produce an overview of the number of replicates etc.:

```
> data( ox )
> ox <- Meth( ox )

The following variables from the data frame
"ox" are used as the Meth variables:
meth: meth
item: item
repl: repl
   y: y
        #Replicates
Method   1   2   3 #Items #Obs: 354 Values:  min  med  max
    CO   1   4  56     61       177         22.2 78.6 93.5
 pulse   1   4  56     61       177         24.0 75.0 94.0
```

We see that we have data on 61 items (children) with three replicates on 56 of them, two replicates on 4 and one replicate on 1 child.

We also see that the values of the measurements range from 22 to 94 – measurements are percentage oxygen saturation.

We can now fit a model with constant bias to the data in the Meth object ox. This is a standard random effects model, and since the replicates are linked, we specify that the item×replicate interaction be included in the model to accommodate this:

```
> m1 <- BA.est( ox, IxR=TRUE )
> m1

Conversion between methods:
               alpha    beta      sd   LoA: lower    upper
To:    From:
CO     CO      0.000   1.000   3.146      -6.293    6.293
       pulse   2.470   1.000   6.169      -9.867   14.808
pulse  CO     -2.470   1.000   6.169     -14.808    9.867
       pulse   0.000   1.000   5.649     -11.298   11.298

Variance components (sd):
          IxR    MxI    res
CO      3.416  2.928  2.225
pulse   3.416  2.928  3.994
```

We see that the conversion from pulse to CO using this model involves adding 2.47, that the prediction standard deviation is 6.17, and that the limits of agreement are $(-14.8, 9.9)\%$.

We now expand the model to allow for non-constant bias, i.e. a linear relationship between the measurement methods. In the first place we use the AltReg function:

```
> m2 <- AltReg( ox, IxR=TRUE, eps=1E-5 )

AltReg converged after  27 iterations
Last convergence criterion was  8.790823e-06

> m2

Conversion between methods:
               alpha    beta      sd
To:    From:
CO     CO      0.000   1.000   2.899
       pulse  -2.257   1.065   6.390
pulse  CO      2.120   0.939   6.002
       pulse   0.000   1.000   5.772

Variance components (sd):
            s.d.
Method     IxR    MxI    res
  CO      3.524  2.979  2.050
  pulse   3.310  2.798  4.081
```

The default output has the same structure as the output from BA.est, but we note that the β for converting between methods is now different from 1; there is a clear slope in the estimates. The difference between methods lies mainly in the residual variances, where the pulse method is the least accurate with a residual standard deviation of 4%, twice that of the CO method.

We get pretty much the same conclusion if we use the BUGS machinery to produce estimates of the variance components. But the output from BUGS will also tell us about the uncertainty of these variance estimates:

```
> m3 <- MCmcmc( ox, IxR=TRUE, n.iter=50000 )

Comparison of 2 methods, using 354 measurements
on 61 items, with up to 3 replicate measurements,
(replicate values are in the set: 1 2 3 )
( 2 * 61 * 3 = 366 ):

No. items with measurements on each method:
        #Replicates
Method  1   2   3 #Items #Obs: 354 Values:  min   med   max
  CO    1   4  56    61      177          22.2 78.6 93.5
  pulse 1   4  56    61      177          24.0 75.0 94.0

Simulation run of a model with
- method by item and item by replicate interaction:
- using 4 chains run for 50000 iterations
  (of which 25000 are burn-in),
- monitoring every 25 values of the chain:
- giving a posterior sample of 4000 observations.

Initializing chain 1: Initializing chain 2: Initializing chain 3:
Initializing chain 4: Sampling has been started...
```

Once the model have been fitted (i.e. we have run the chains sufficiently long according to our own prejudice), we can get results in the same form as those from BA.est or AltReg by applying the function MethComp:

```
> MethComp( m3 )

Conversion between methods:
              alpha   beta     sd
To:   From:
CO    CO      0.000  1.000  2.435
      pulse  -6.131  1.117  5.081
pulse CO       5.489  0.895  4.544
      pulse   0.000  1.000  6.015

Variance components (sd):
```

```
         s.d.
Method    IxR   MxI    res
  CO     3.795 3.197 1.722
  pulse  3.383 2.860 4.253
```

The results are close to those obtained by the `AltReg` function, although the parameters of the conversion line look somewhat different. The similarity is apparent from the plot in Figure 7.3.

The MCMC approach gives more detail if we use the default listing of the `MCmcmc` object which includes the posterior credible intervals:

```
> m3
```

```
Conversion between methods:
              alpha   beta     sd
To:    From:
CO     CO      0.000  1.000  2.435
       pulse  -6.131  1.117  5.081
pulse  CO      5.489  0.895  4.544
       pulse   0.000  1.000  6.015


Variance components (sd):
         s.d.
Method    IxR   MxI    res
  CO     3.795 3.197 1.722
  pulse  3.383 2.860 4.253


Variance components with 95 % cred.int.:
    method   CO                   pulse
     qnt    50%  2.5% 97.5%    50%  2.5% 97.5%
SD
IxR        3.795 3.032 4.556 3.383 2.751 4.069
MxI        3.197 2.358 4.276 2.860 2.091 3.811
res        1.722 0.246 2.791 4.253 3.601 4.995
tot        5.281 4.608 6.108 6.172 5.526 6.906


Mean parameters with 95 % cred.int.:
                  50%     2.5%  97.5% P(>0/1)
alpha[pulse.CO]   5.485  -3.112 13.411  0.904
alpha[CO.pulse]  -6.135 -16.965  3.063  0.096
beta[pulse.CO]    0.895   0.791  1.007  0.034
beta[CO.pulse]    1.117   0.993  1.264  0.966
```

```
Note that intercepts in conversion formulae are adjusted to get
conversion formulae that represent the same line both ways,
and hence the median intercepts in the posterior do not agree
exactly with those given in the conversion formulae.
```

The slope of the conversion line between the methods is actually different from 1 (1 is right at one end of the 95% credible interval for β), but it is also clear from this that the residual standard deviation of the CO method is quite poorly determined, which may explain the

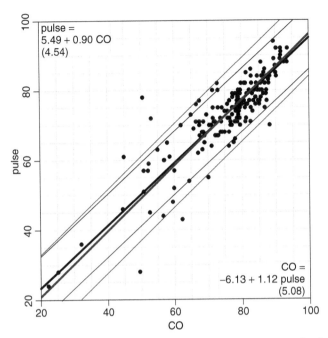

Figure 7.3   Estimated conversion between the two methods of measuring oxygen saturation. The black line and black text are based on the posterior medians from a Monte Carlo chain simulation. The blue lines (please see color plate section) are based on the estimates from the alternating regressions procedure.

rather narrower prediction intervals obtained from the MCMC procedure. Using the posterior median seems a bit optimistic – there are 177 points in the display, so the 95% prediction intervals should miss about 9 of them; but the MCMC-based interval misses rather more (see Figure 7.3).

```
> par( mar=c(3,3,1,1), mgp=c(3,1,0)/1.6, xaxs="i", yaxs="i" )
> plot.MCmcmc( m3, axlim=c(20,100), grid=seq(20,100,5) )
> par(new=TRUE)
> plot.MethComp( m2, axlim=c(20,100), eqn=FALSE, col.lines="blue",
+                points=TRUE, pch=16, grid=FALSE )
```

```
Note:
 Replicate measurements are taken as separate items!
```

We now take a look at the posterior distribution of the variance component estimates from the four chains we ran:

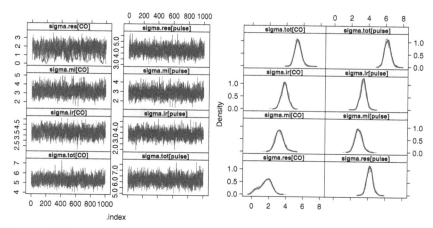

Figure 7.4   Monitoring of the posterior distributions of the estimates of the variance components from the oximetry data.

```
> print( trace.MCmcmc( m3, "sd" ) )

> print( post.MCmcmc( m3, "sd" ) )
```

As seen in Figure 7.4, there is some instability in the simulation from one or two of the chains, both from the trace plot and from the plot of the smoothed posteriors from each of the chains. This is a reflection of the general phenomenon that estimation of variance components requires large sample sizes. In summary, it seems safe to use the conversion equation and corresponding prediction limits provided by the BUGS output as shown in Figure 7.3. A little more reluctance is required to use the posterior distributions of the variances for construction of confidence intervals. However, this is all we have; using various approximations for the distribution of the maximum likelihood estimates variance components seems even more dubious.

7.6   Models with non-constant variance

The extensions presented in this section, with its profusion of formulae, are not really worth pursuing. This material is included for the sake of completeness.

The general model (7.1) assumes that the random effect terms have constant variances, i.e. the variance only depends on method. However, it would be natural to allow the variation to depend on covariates (other than method) or on the actual level of the measurement. The former will normally depend on the subject-matter, whereas the latter is a possibility that routinely should be explored.

7.6.1   Linear dependence of residual standard error

A straightforward extension of model (7.1) would be

$$e_{mir} \sim \mathcal{N}(0, (\sigma_m + \zeta_m \mu_i)^2), \qquad \text{s.d.}(e_{mir}) = \sigma_m + \zeta_m \mu_i,$$

i.e. letting the measurement standard deviation depend linearly on the 'true' value μ_i. This will have the effect that the resulting prediction limits will be straight lines. Model (7.1) corresponds to setting $\zeta_m = 0$. Similar specifications could of course also be implemented for the other variance components.

However, there is also an overparametrization in this specification; a transformation $\mu_i \mapsto \xi_i = \gamma + \delta\mu_i$ will give the specification

$$\text{s.d.}(e_{mir}) = \sigma_m + \zeta_m \mu_i = \sigma_m + \zeta_m (\xi_i - \gamma)/\delta$$
$$= (\sigma_m - \gamma/\delta) + (\zeta_m/\delta)\xi_i.$$

This is in principle the same phenomenon as with the mean specification. For two specifications of the model,

$$y_{mir} = \alpha_m + \beta_m(\mu_i + a_i) + c_{mi} + e_{mir}, \qquad \text{s.d.}(e_{mir}) = \sigma_m + \zeta_m \mu_i,$$
$$y_{mir} = \tilde{\alpha}_m + \tilde{\beta}_m(\xi_i + a_i) + c_{mi} + e_{mir}, \qquad \text{s.d.}(e_{mir}) = \tilde{\sigma}_m + \tilde{\zeta}_m \mu_i,$$

the parameters will be linked by

$$\xi_i = \gamma + \delta\mu_i,$$
$$\tilde{\alpha}_m = \alpha_m - \beta_m \gamma/\delta,$$
$$\tilde{\beta}_m = \beta_m/\delta,$$
$$\tilde{\sigma}_m = \sigma_m - \zeta_m \gamma/\delta,$$
$$\tilde{\zeta}_m = \zeta_m/\delta.$$

Since the standard deviations of the random effects are part of the prediction equations we must find out what standard deviation we should use for a given value of y_{m0}. If we use the previous derivation of the conversion formulae, we have

$$y_{10} = \alpha_1 + \beta_1(\mu_0 + a_0) + c_{10} + e_{10}$$

$$\Rightarrow \quad \mu_0 + a_0 = \frac{y_{10} - \alpha_1 - c_{10} - e_{10}}{\beta_1}$$

and hence the prediction

$$y_{2|1} = \alpha_2 + \beta_2(\mu_0 + a_0) + c_{20} + e_{20}$$

$$= \alpha_2 + \beta_2 \frac{y_{10} - \alpha_1 - c_{10} - e_{10}}{\beta_1} + c_{20} + e_{20}$$

$$= \alpha_{2|1} + \beta_{2|1} y_{01} - \beta_{2|1}(c_{10} + e_{10}) + c_{20} + e_{20},$$

where $\beta_{2|1} = \beta_2/\beta_1$ and $\alpha_{2|1} = \alpha_2 - \beta_{2|1}\alpha_1$. As noted in Section 7.3, these two quantities are invariant under the changes in parameters induced by a linear transformation of the μ_is.

The variance of the prediction y_{20} based on an observation of y_{10} is

$$\mathrm{var}(y_{2|1}) = \beta_{2|1}^2 \left(\tau_1^2 + (\sigma_1 + \zeta_1\mu_0)^2\right) + \left(\tau_2^2 + (\sigma_2 + \zeta_2\mu_0)^2\right).$$

This can only be applied if we have a useful estimate of μ_0. The only plausible estimate is the mean from the equation defining y_{10}, i.e. $\hat{\mu}_0 = (y_{10} - \alpha_1)/\beta_1$, so a reasonable estimate for $\mathrm{var}(y_{2|1})$ is

$$\mathrm{var}(y_{2|1}) = \beta_{2|1}^2 \left(\tau_1^2 + (\sigma_1 + \zeta_1(y_{10} - \alpha_1)/\beta_1)^2\right)$$
$$+ \left(\tau_2^2 + (\sigma_2 + \zeta_2(y_{10} - \alpha_1)/\beta_1)^2\right).$$

In the alternative parametrization induced by $\mu_i \mapsto \xi_i = \gamma + \delta\mu_i$ we get

$$\mathrm{var}(y_{2|1}) = \beta_{2|1}^2 \left(\tau_1^2 + (\tilde{\sigma}_1 + \tilde{\zeta}_1(y_{10} - \tilde{\alpha}_1)/\tilde{\beta}_1)^2\right)$$
$$+ \left(\tau_2^2 + (\tilde{\sigma}_2 + \tilde{\zeta}_2(y_{10} - \tilde{\alpha}_1)/\tilde{\beta}_1)^2\right).$$

But this is the same as above because

$$\tilde{\sigma}_1 + \tilde{\zeta}_1(y_{10} - \tilde{\alpha}_1)/\tilde{\beta}_1 = \sigma_1 - \zeta_1\gamma/\delta + \zeta_1/\delta\frac{y_{10} - (\alpha_1 - \beta_1\gamma/\delta)}{\beta_1/\delta}$$

$$= \sigma_1 - \zeta_1\gamma/\delta + \zeta_1\left(y_{10} - (\alpha_1 - \beta_1\gamma/\delta)\right)/\beta_1$$

$$= \sigma_1 + \zeta_1(y_{10} - \alpha_1)/\beta_1.$$

Hence, with the given specification of the variance, the model is invariant under linear transformation of the μ_is, and the prediction interval can safely be derived from the posterior samples as the only instability in these is due to the linear indetermination of the parameters, which has no effect on the parameters of interest.

However, as was pointed out in Section 4.7, the prediction limits for conversion between methods cannot be represented by the same lines in a plot – limits that are symmetric and increasing for prediction of y_2 from y_1 will not be symmetric when read the other way round. Suppose methods are related by

$$y_{mir} = \alpha_m + \beta_m(\mu_i + a_i) + c_{mi} + e_{mir}, \qquad (7.4)$$

$$\text{s.d.}(a_{ir}) = \omega, \quad \text{s.d.}(c_{mi}) = \tau_m, \quad \text{s.d.}(e_{mir}) = \sigma_m + \zeta_m\mu_i.$$

A worked example using a fictitious set of parameters is shown in Figure 7.5. The parameters used were as follows:

method	α	β	τ	σ	ζ
1	0.0	1.0	0.3	0.3	0.05
2	2.0	1.2	0.3	0.4	0.08

It is clear how the prediction intervals are different in the two directions. There is of course nothing wrong with this, but it would be an intuitively appealing property to be able to show both predictions using one set of limits.

There is currently no estimation method for models where the standard deviation of the random effects depends on the mean. Hence, it seems that the only feasible way to go about analysis of a data set

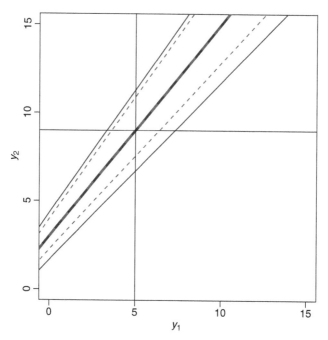

Figure 7.5   Example of prediction limits when the relationship between methods is as in equation (7.4). The blue lines refer to the prediction of y_2 from y_1 and the dotted red lines to the predictions the other way round (please see color plate section).

with non-constant variances is to try to transform the measurements to a scale where the variances *are* constant. This is detailed in the next chapter.

7.7   Summary

When two or more methods of measurement are compared, and it has been established that the bias is not constant, then proceed as follows:

1. Draw Bland–Altman plots to check whether the variance is constant over the range of measurements.

2. If variances vary over the range of observation, find a transformation that renders the variance constant.

3. Fit the appropriate model using either alternating regressions or BUGS.
   Remember to include the item×replicate effect if replicates are linked.
   If more than three methods are compared, consider whether the method×item effect should have method-specific variances or not.

4. Report the conversion equations between all pairs of methods with prediction limits, preferably in the form of graphs.

5. Report the estimated variance components, preferably with confidence intervals, either from bootstrapping or some MCMC-based estimation procedure.

8

Transformation of measurements

If a simple Bland–Altman plot of differences versus averages between methods shows signs of non-constant variance, one possible way of compensating for this heteroscedasticity is to find a suitable data transformation that stabilizes the variance. There may, however, also be instances where we want a transformation of the measurement data from a purely substantive point of view. It is normally only the log transformation that is mentioned in the literature, because this is the only transformation that gives an immediately understandable interpretation: differences between logarithms are logarithms of ratios and therefore there is a simple back-transform of the differences of the logarithms to a clinically meaningful scale – the ratios.

This is one reason for taking the approach based on limits of agreement a step further to actual calibration/prediction, because prediction equations derived between methods on a transformed scale can be graphically back-transformed to the original scale, thus bypassing the problems of back-transforming differences to something clinically meaningful. This means that the relationship between methods is not reported in analytical form, but only graphically in the form of a chart converting between the measurement methods.

Comparing Clinical Measurement Methods: A Practical Guide   Bendix Carstensen
© 2010 John Wiley & Sons, Ltd

Once the conversion plot is drawn, it can of course be rotated 45° to resemble a traditional Bland–Altman plot. The only difference will be that the limits of agreement are no longer horizontal lines, but more general curves. To my knowledge this approach was first proposed by Lise Brøndsted in her PhD dissertation [9].

8.1   Log transformation

When the variance is increasing with the measurement values, the first remedy is to transform the original data by the log. In the simplest case with two methods and one measurement by each, the limits of agreement will be transformed back to limits of agreement on the ratio scale, i.e. expressing the limits of agreement for the ratio of method 1 to method 2 – as a function of the geometric mean, to be absolutely correct.

8.2   Transformations of percentages

For measurements whose values are fractions (or percentages) with a well-defined upper and lower boundary, differences between methods will naturally be smaller toward the ends of the scale. For percentages it would be natural to use one of the classical link functions used for binomial data, the logit or (complementary) log-minus-log. These have the drawback that the differences on the transformed scales are not easily interpreted in clinical terms, so the classical reporting of the simple (constant bias) model via limits of agreement is not feasible. The model should instead be used to construct a conversion line between methods with prediction limits on the transformed scale. This can then be transformed back to the original scale in the form of a plot that gives prediction intervals between the methods on the original (clinically relevant) scale. These will of course not be straight lines as illustrated in the next worked example.

8.2.1   A worked example

By way of illustration we give a worked example of comparing measurements that are inherently percentages. We use the oximetry data collected at the Royal Children's Hospital in Melbourne, introduced in Chapter 2, p. 47.

Since the measurements are percentages, it would be natural to apply a transformation to the data that reflects the fact that observations are necessarily between 0 and 100%. One natural choice is the logit transformation

$$z = \log\left(\frac{y}{100 - y}\right).$$

From Figure 8.1 it is evident that the variance of the measurements is diminishing toward 100%, and that this is largely remedied by applying the logit transform.

Once we have made this transformation we can fit the simple model (5.2) with constant bias:

$$y_{mir} = \alpha_m + a_{ir} + c_{mi} + e_{mir}, \quad \text{var}(a_{ir}) = \omega^2, \quad \text{var}(c_{mi}) = \tau_m^2,$$

$$\text{var}(e_{mir}) = \sigma_m^2.$$

The two values of τ cannot be separated since we only have two methods (see Chapter 5). Fitting the variance component model gives a mean bias of $\hat{\alpha} = \text{pulse} - \text{CO} = -0.1564$ and variance components

$$\tau_{CO} = 0.157,$$

$$\tau_{pulse} = 0.157,$$

$$\omega = 0.221,$$

$$\sigma_{CO} = 0.160,$$

$$\sigma_{pulse} = 0.179.$$

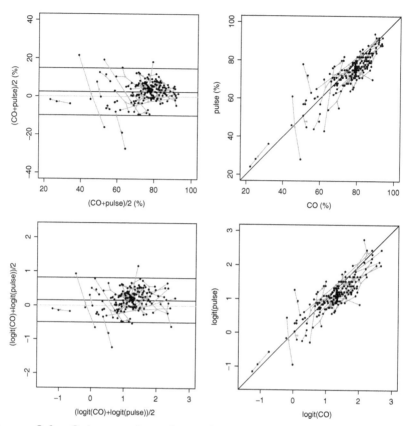

Figure 8.1   Oximetry data from the Royal Children's Hospital in Melbourne. The linked measurements for each child are indicated in gray with lines to the mean of all three measurements. The top plots are on the original scale, the bottom ones are logit-transformed data.

These estimates give limits of agreement (on the logit scale)

$$\hat{\alpha} \pm 2\sqrt{\tau_{CO}^2 + \tau_{pulse}^2 + \sigma_{CO}^2 + \sigma_{pulse}^2} = (-0.811, 0.498),$$

or the relationship between logits,

$$\text{logit(pulse)} = \text{logit(CO)} + 0.156 \pm 2 \times 0.327 \qquad (8.1)$$

$$\Updownarrow$$

$$\text{OR}_{\text{pulse vs. CO}} = e^{-0.156} \overset{\times}{\div} e^{0.654} = 0.85 \overset{\times}{\div} 1.92.$$

It would be difficult to use this directly, since odds ratios of saturation percentages are not readily understood in the clinic. However, the relation is easily transformed and plotted on the original scale:

1. Generate a sequence of CO values, say from 20 to 100 in steps of 0.1, and make a logit transform of these.

2. Use equation (8.1) to generate predicted values of logit(pulse) with prediction limits.

3. Back-transform these to the original pulse scale and plot against the originally generated sequence of CO-values.

This will give a plot that is applicable for conversion between the two methods, but based on a model fitted on the transformed scale, as shown in Figure 8.2.

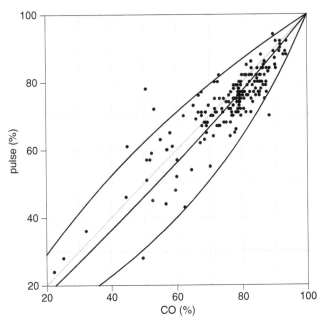

Figure 8.2   Oximetry data from the Royal Children's Hospital in Melbourne. The 95% prediction limits between the methods are derived from a model for logit-transformed data.

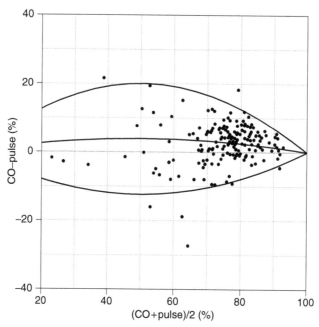

Figure 8.3   Oximetry data from the Royal Children's Hospital in Melbourne. The 95% limits of agreement between the methods are derived from a model for logit-transformed data, assuming constant difference on the logit scale.

This conversion plot can be rotated 45° by taking the computed coordinates of the points (y_{CO}, y_{pulse}) and replacing them by $\left(y_{CO} - y_{pulse}, (y_{CO} + y_{pulse})/2\right)$ to give a plot of the limits of agreement as illustrated in Figure 8.3.

8.2.2   Implementation in MethComp

The transformation of measurement values is an external thing relative to the models and procedures presented in this book; transformation is applied first, the relevant model fitted to the transformed data, and in the reporting the back-transform is applied to the plot.

This has been implemented in the MethComp package for R via an argument to the functions BA.est, AltReg and MCmcmc. The transformation is obeyed by the plot methods, so that back-transformed plots are shown, using the original measurement scale.

8.3   Other transformations

The example above used the logit transformation for data which were recorded as fractions. But there was nothing in the example that relied on anything but the monotonicity of the transformation. Thus any arbitrary transformation that can remedy variance inhomogeneity and/or non-linearity will be applicable to produce a plot converting from one method to another and/or the corresponding Bland–Altman plot. However, the latter is only relevant if the two methods actually do measure on the same scale – otherwise differences between measurements by the two methods have no meaning.

Furthermore, there is no reason why the transformation applied to both methods should be the same. It will just imply that the back-transformation to the original scale is different for different methods.

8.4   Several methods

If more than two methods are compared we may in principle select different transformations in order to make relations linear with constant variances. Once the analysis and conversion equations have been derived on the transformed scales, we can make a back-transformation to the original measurement scales for each pair of methods.

8.5   Variance components

The major problem with the transformation approach is that we get estimates of the variance components (i.e. the standard deviations) on the transformed scale. Since the transformed scale is where the models are fitted, this is where the variance components can be discussed. Thus the variance components will not in general have any direct interpretation and in reality only be of interest in comparing the precision of the methods.

If we have chosen the same transformation for all methods it will be possible to compare the variance components between methods, otherwise not. For this reason it is generally advisable to choose the same transformation for all methods if possible.

8.6   Summary

If it turns out that the variance of the differences between methods varies with the level of measurement, proceed as follows:

1. Transform the measurements so that differences between methods have uniform variance.

2. Do the appropriate analysis on the transformed scale, including derivation of the conversion equations with prediction limits.

3. Report the conversion equations graphically by back-transforming the conversions to the original measurement scale(s).

4. The relative merits of the methods in terms of the variance components must be evaluated on the transformed scale.

9

Repeatability, reproducibility and coefficient of variation

The aim of a method comparison study is not just to derive the limits of agreement or mean conversion between methods; the assessment of method-specific repeatability and reproducibility is of interest in its own right. Repeatability and reproducibility can only be assessed when replicate measurements by each method are available.

If the standard deviation of a measurement by method m attributable to measurement error is σ_m, the repeatability/reproducibility coefficient is defined as the upper prediction limit for the absolute difference of two measurements by the same method, that is $1.96 \times \sqrt{2}\,\sigma_m = 2.77\,\sigma_m$. The distinction between repeatability and reproducibility is only a question of the sources of variation included in the definition of σ [17].

If replicate measurements by a method are available, it is simple to estimate the measurement error for a method, using a model with fixed effect of item (person), and then taking the residual standard deviation as the measurement error standard deviation. But if replicates are linked this may produce an overestimate (see Chapter 8, p. 47).

Comparing Clinical Measurement Methods: A Practical Guide   Bendix Carstensen
© 2010 John Wiley & Sons, Ltd

9.1 Repeatability

The repeatability coefficient (or simply repeatability) for a method is defined as the upper limit of a prediction interval for the absolute difference between two measurements by the same method on the same item under *identical* circumstances – essentially by the same operator in the same laboratory on the same day [17].

Consider the general model for observations from a method comparison study:

$$y_{mir} = \alpha_m + \beta_m (\mu_i + a_{ir} + c_{mi}) + e_{mir},$$

$$a_{ir} \sim \mathcal{N}(0, \omega^2), \quad c_{mi} \sim \mathcal{N}(0, \tau_m^2), \quad e_{mir} \sim \mathcal{N}(0, \sigma_m^2),$$

The variation between measurements under identical circumstances for a particular method m must of course include the variance component σ_m.

The method by item variance, τ_m^2, refers to the part of the method×item variation not explained by the term $\beta_m \mu_i$; the random effects (c_{mi}) are constant across replicates, so they play no role in evaluating the repeatability, hence τ_m should *not* be included.

Whether the item×replicate variation, ω, should be considered or not depends on the circumstances of the particular experiment conducted. ω represents the variation of the 'true' value $(\mu_i + a_{ir})$ *within* item, between replicates. So if replicates are exchangeable within methods, this effect will not be in the model, but it will be included in the estimate of σ_m, to the extent that a replication scheme can be constructed. It may therefore be argued that in the case of an experiment with linked replicates, the relevant quantity to use for constructing the repeatability coefficient is always $\sqrt{\beta_m^2 \omega^2 + \sigma_m^2}$. However, if the variation between replicates within item is irrelevant for the repeatability, the component $\beta_m^2 \omega^2$ should not be included. This would, for example, be the case if replicates were taken with rather large time intervals and at different times for different items, so that experimental conditions between replicates could not be considered 'identical' in the sense mentioned in the ISO standard [17]. So the between-replicates variation should only be taken as part of the reproducibility if replicates are so closely spaced that they can be considered as taken under 'identical' circumstances.

By the same token, the repeatability is only estimable from an experiment with exchangeable replicates if *all* measurements on the same item (by all methods) can be considered as taken under 'identical' circumstances. In this case the residual variation includes the variation between replicates, even though the latter is not separately estimable. If the exchangeable replicates cannot be assumed to be taken under identical circumstances, we have a situation where the variation between replicates must be excluded, but where it is impossible by design to separate it from the residual variation, and hence the repeatability is not estimable from the experiment at hand.

So even if the variance component representing the variation between replicates is not included in the model for experiments with exchangeable replicates, it does not mean that it is non-existent (i.e. equal to 0), but merely that it is inseparable by design from the residual variation σ_m.

In summary:

- If replicates are exchangeable, and replication instances can be regarded as fulfilling the repeatability conditions, the residual variation σ_m can be used as a basis for calculation of repeatability. The estimate of σ_m from the general model will be indistinguishable from the estimate of the residual standard deviation obtained using only using data from method m in a model with item alone.

- If replicates are linked, the variation between replicates is captured by the item×replicate variance component ω. If replicates fulfill the repeatability conditions, the variation in measurement standard deviation is estimated from the general model by $\sqrt{\beta_m^2 \omega^2 + \sigma_m^2}$, otherwise as σ_m.

Heuristically speaking, when replicates are linked, measurements by other methods contain essential information required to estimate the residual variation; if replicates are exchangeable, they do not.

9.2   Reproducibility

The reproducibility coefficient for a method is defined as the upper limits of a prediction interval for the absolute difference between two measurements by the same method on the same item under *different* circumstances, normally referring to different laboratories. This is a topic that is not covered by the types of studies considered in this book.

There may be circumstances where 'methods' are synonymous with laboratories, and where the experiment aims to quantify the repeatability for each laboratory as well as providing conversion formulae between measurements taken at different laboratories. But this approach explicitly takes the laboratories as fixed effects (the methods are *specific* laboratories), whereas reproducibility addresses the variation between (*randomly* selected) laboratories. So if different laboratories are not involved in the original experimental design, then there is no way to get a handle on the between-laboratory variation – the reproducibility.

If different (randomly selected) laboratories are represented as a further layer of replication on top of within-laboratory replicates, both repeatability and reproducibility can of course be estimated, even separately for each method. This would require an extension of the models presented in this book. In practice it would, however, be rare to see method comparison (which addresses an intra-laboratory question) mixed up with estimation of reproducibility (which addresses an inter-laboratory question).

9.3   Coefficient of variation

The precision of a measurement method is often given as the coefficient of variation (CV). The CV is not something to consider in addition to the sources of variation already discussed in this book, but rather a question of choice of the scale on which to report the measurement variation.

Formally, the coefficient of variation of a variable is the standard deviation divided by the mean, $CV = \sigma/\mu$. If we are considering measurements with different means, but constant coefficient of variation, we have, for different observations y_j with mean μ_j and standard deviation σ_j,

$$CV = \sigma_j/\mu_j \quad \Leftrightarrow \quad \sigma_j = CV \times \mu_j.$$

So the assumption of a constant coefficient of variation amounts to an assumption that the standard deviation is proportional to the mean. Which, since $\mu_j = CV/\sigma_j$, implies that measurements necessarily are positive.

In the case of measurement methods the CV is a relevant quantity when the standard deviation is assumed to be proportional to the measurement itself. This would imply that prediction intervals would be of the form $\mu \pm 2 \times CV\mu$, assuming a normal distribution of errors. Clearly, when measurements are positive this is only sensible when the coefficient of variation is less than 0.5; otherwise the lower bound of the prediction interval would be negative – clearly not meaningful for measurements that by definition only assume positive values.

However, the upper limit of 0.5 for the CV is a rather arbitrary limit as well; it would be different if we were using 90% or 99% prediction intervals.

The snag is elsewhere. If the measurement error is assumed proportional to the mean, we are essentially assuming a multiplicative structure for the errors; the error is a multiple of the mean (the 'true' measurement). It would therefore be natural to assume (or require) that prediction intervals were multiplicative in the sense that the upper and lower limits were obtained by multiplying and dividing the estimated mean by the same factor.

Consequently, we should not be using the additive scale for constructing prediction intervals, but the multiplicative. This means that we assume an additive structure for errors on the log scale. Hence, the multiplicative structure can be obtained by assuming a normal model for the log-transformed data – the normality is mainly used to justify the prediction intervals of the form $\mu \pm 2\sigma$.

Conveniently, it turns out that after log-transforming data, the standard deviations can be interpreted as coefficients of variation. Suppose a variable Y has mean μ and standard deviation σ. Then by the δ-rule,

$$\text{s.d. }(\log(Y)) \approx \sigma \times \left.\frac{d\log(y)}{dy}\right|_{y=\mu} = \sigma/\mu = CV.$$

Thus, if we can assume that the mean and the standard deviation of the variable are both constant in a sample, the coefficient of variation can be estimated by the standard deviation of the log-transformed variable. If both mean and standard deviation vary across the sample, we may assume that they are constant in smaller chunks of the material, and use the log transformation to estimate the CV in each chunk. If we additionally assume that the CV is constant (i.e. that the standard deviation is proportional to the mean), we do not need to subdivide the material into smaller chunks – we can just estimate the CV as the residual standard deviation from a suitable model for the log-transformed data. And the assumption of constant CV now merely is an assumption of constant standard deviation of the log-transformed data, which can be checked in the usual way by regressing the absolute residuals on the means.

9.3.1   Symmetric interval on the log scale

The relevant quantities in constructing prediction intervals on the original measurement scale are the multiplicative factors of the form $\exp(2\sigma)$, where σ is the relevant prediction standard deviation on the log scale. If σ is small (less than 0.05, say), $\exp(2\sigma) \approx (1 + 2\sigma)$, so we can use the approximations

$$\mu \overset{\times}{\div} \exp(2\sigma) \approx \mu \overset{\times}{\div} (1 + 2\sigma) \approx \mu \pm 2\sigma\mu. \tag{9.1}$$

But if σ is substantially larger than 0.05, these approximations will be inaccurate, and the only relevant way of constructing the prediction intervals will be by using a multiplicative factor, as in the left-hand side of (9.1).

So in all cases where the coefficient of variation is of relevance, it should be reported as the standard deviation for the log-transformed data, and preferably also the multiplicative factor $\exp(2\sigma)$ for constructing prediction intervals should be given.

In conclusion, the coefficient of variation is just a way of reporting results for log-transformed data. Of course it is only relevant to do so if errors are actually proportional to the means, i.e. if the normal model fits the log-transformed data.

The coefficient of variation should always be given as the standard deviation from the log-transformed data; if it is small (less than 5%)

it will coincide with the traditionally computed CV; if it is larger the traditionally computed CV is not a useful measure – but the standard deviation of the log-transformed data is.

9.3.2   Computing the CV correctly

As an aside, it should be mentioned that the standard deviation of data transformed by the natural logarithm is always computable, whereas replicate measurements are required to compute the coefficient of variation as the standard deviation divided by the mean. If replicate measurements are not available, there is no way to get a handle on the variance for different means.

The variation used to estimate the CV based on log-transformed data is the *residual* variation derived using some model for the mean value. If this model just specifies a common mean for all observations, we actually *do* have replicate measurements (all observations are replicates of the same), and hence the two methods of estimation will roughly coincide.

Occasionally, the overall residual standard deviation is just divided by the overall mean and used as estimate of the CV. This is inherently nonsensical since estimates from a model assuming constant mean and standard deviation are used to provide estimates in a model assuming the standard deviation to be proportional to the (varying) mean. Alternatively, the underlying argument could be that the CV of the variable in this particular population is computed, i.e. a population parameter and hence a quantity totally unrelated to the method precision.

If the range of the measurements is fairly small (i.e. the ratio of the largest to the smallest measurement is 2 or less), this erroneous method will, however, give a pretty good estimate of the CV, but this is merely due to the fact that such data really do not allow discrimination between a model with constant standard deviation and a model with standard deviation proportional to the mean.

9.3.3   Transformations

Using the log-transformed data to estimate the CV of course comes at a price, namely that whatever mean value structure we are assuming (in this book, a linear relationship between measurement methods) is assumed to be on the log-scale too.

This raises the more general issue of data transformation prior to data analysis. Two principles can be invoked:

1. Choose a transformation that provides the best fit to data.

2. Choose a transformation that makes subject-matter sense.

The first choice is always possible; for example, there are methods available for choosing from a family of parametrized transformations (such as the Box–Cox family). The second choice is only possible if some prior knowledge of the measurements is available, but it has the advantage that the results from the fitted model are more easily interpretable.

The practical aspects of data transformation are discussed further in Chapter 8.

10

Measures of association and agreement

A number of summary measures describing the agreement between methods have been proposed in the literature. Most of these are (intended to be) scale-free in the sense that the absolute scale of measurement does not enter into the measure. This seems to be an attempt to define a purely statistical machinery for comparing methods. That limits the applicability of such measures, since assessment of methods without sound clinical judgment is bound to be error-prone. Some pressure for purely statistical procedures comes from (a subset of the) clinicians who dearly want to get an 'answer' instead of relevant input as a basis for clinical decisions, as the latter are always unpleasant and troublesome to make.

One particular drawback of summary measures is the inherent assumption that the agreement is constant over the range of measurement, i.e. that the bias and the variance components are constant. Of course one could argue that the summary was a weighted average of the biases and variances, but that would necessarily require some assumption about the distribution of the 'true' measurements.

Comparing Clinical Measurement Methods: A Practical Guide   Bendix Carstensen
© 2010 John Wiley & Sons, Ltd

10.1   Individual bioequivalence criterion

The US Food and Drug Administration [16] have proposed to compare the mean squared difference between a test (T) and a reference (R) drug to the mean squared difference between replicate measurements of the reference drug $(R$ and $R')$. The individual bioequivalence criterion (IBC) was detailed by Barnhart et al. [5] as

$$\text{IBC} = \frac{E(Y_{iT} - Y_{iR})^2 - E(Y_{iR} - Y_{iR'})^2}{E(Y_{iR} - Y_{iR'})^2/2},$$

where Y_{iT} is the measurement for individual i by method T (test method). This is rewritten in Barnhart's notation as

$$\text{IBC} = \frac{(\mu_t - \mu_R)^2 + \sigma_D^2 + \sigma_{WT}^2 - \sigma_{WR}^2}{\sigma_{WR}^2},$$

where σ_{WT}^2 and σ_{WR}^2 are the residual variances for the test and reference methods and σ_D the variance of the differences between methods, i.e. the 'subject by formulation interaction variance'.

Note that the IBC is only relevant to compute in a model with constant bias between methods, since it is a summary measure. If the bias or the variances are not constant, the measure depends on the 'true' value of the quantity measured.

If we use the general model (7.1) from Chapter 7 (since we must use a model with constant bias), and assume that method 1 is the reference method, we get

$$y_{mir} = \alpha_m + \mu_i + a_{ir} + c_{mi} + e_{mir}. \tag{10.1}$$

If we assume that the comparison between the reference method and the test method are from different replicates, i.e. are not assumed taken at the same time point or similar, we get

$$E(y_{1ir} - y_{2is})^2 = E(\alpha_1 - \alpha_2 + a_{ir} - a_{is} + c_{1i} - c_{2i} + e_{1ir} - e_{2is})^2$$
$$= (\alpha_1 - \alpha_2)^2 + 2\omega^2 + \tau_1^2 + \tau_2^2 + \sigma_1^2 + \sigma_2^2$$

and

$$E(y_{1ir} - y_{1is})^2 = E(a_{ir} - a_{is} + e_{1ir} - e_{2is})^2 = 2\omega^2 + 2\sigma_1^2,$$

and hence, in the notation of this book,

$$IBC = \frac{(\alpha_1 - \alpha_2)^2 + \tau_1^2 + \tau_2^2 + \sigma_2^2 - \sigma_1^2}{\omega^2 + \sigma_1^2}.$$

Thus we see that if we have data from an experiment with linked replicates (i.e. where we have the random effects a_{ir} in the model) we must take the variance of these into account, i.e. the between-replicates variation must be included with the residual variation of the reference method. This requires that the way the linked replicates are made is meaningful in terms of generalizability to future situations.

However, it might be of relevance to consider the IBC as a measure of the extra variability by replacing the reference method 1 by the test method 2 under exactly the same circumstances. Conceptually this is a little odd, since the between-replicates variability is ignored for the comparison between methods, whereas it is included in the assessment of the within-method variability. Therefore it would be more sensible to exclude the between-replicate variation altogether, referring to the hypothetical situation where replicates are taken under exactly identical circumstances, leading to the expression

$$IBC = \frac{(\alpha_1 - \alpha_2)^2 + \tau_1^2 + \tau_2^2 + \sigma_2^2 - \sigma_1^2}{\sigma_1^2}.$$

Either way the IBC compares the residual variation ('pure' measurement error) for method 1 with the extra variation incurred by a switch to method 2, which has three components:

1. $\sigma_2^2 - \sigma_1^2$, the extra (or lesser!) measurement error.

2. $\tau_1^2 + \tau_2^2$, the person by method interactions. Note that this implicitly assumes that the item interaction with the reference method is either negligible or an effect that it is desirable to have with the measurements.

3. $(\alpha_1 - \alpha_2)^2$, the squared bias. Note that this exploits the definition of a reference method; the reference method is unbiased, so we implicitly assume that the squared difference here is solely attributable to the test method.

If replicates are not linked in the observation plan, we may of course still consider model (10.1) but the variance between replicates would then be totally confounded with the residual variance of the reference method, and hence in the practical estimation included with the estimate of σ_1.

The IBC has the appealing property that it shows the 'extra variability' incurred by replacing the reference method by the (new) test method.

10.2   Agreement index

Shao and Zhong [20] defined an agreement index symmetrical in the two methods:

$$\delta = \frac{E[E(x - y|z)]^2}{E[var(x - y|z)]},$$

i.e. the ratio of the mean squared error of $x - y$ to the variance of $x - y$, where x and y are the measurements by the two methods, respectively.

The z in the conditioning is the 'true' value of the measurement, i.e. μ in the notation of this book. This index again implicitly assumes that the bias between the two methods is constant. If this is not the case, the empirical distribution of the zs will be used in computing the outer expectations, even if this distribution is utterly irrelevant. The distribution is of course redundant if the bias is constant, so the outer expectation is either superfluous or misleading.

Assuming a model such as (10.1) or (7.1), i.e. that bias and variance are independent of μ, we have that

$$\delta = \frac{E(x - y)^2}{var(x - y)} = \frac{E(y_{1ir} - y_{2ir})^2}{var(y_{1ir} - y_{2ir})} = \frac{(\alpha_1 - \alpha_2)^2 + \tau_1^2 + \tau_2^2 + \sigma_1^2 + \sigma_2^2}{\tau_1^2 + \tau_2^2 + \sigma_1^2 + \sigma_2^2}.$$

Note that here we have omitted the variance component for the item by replicate effect because we are referring to a situation where we assume that we use the same replicates from different methods.

We could of course also define the measure as referring to different replication occasions, in which case we would get an extra $2\omega^2$ term in both numerator and denominator.

Either way, the δ is merely a measure that summarizes the location and the width of the limits of agreement in one number. Whether this further reduction of the limits of agreement adds anything is doubtful, but it is certainly not an agreement index, since two methods with small bias but very large variances (τs and σs) can produce an index close to 1.

Thus the index displays whether the bias is large relative to the variance, which has little to do with agreement. In the absence of a reference method and the presence of a strong desire to compute some summary measure, it would seem more natural to compute the IBC both ways between the two methods.

10.3   Relative variance index

Shao and Zhong [20] also propose a comparison index for the variances, namely,

$$\tau = \frac{E[\text{var}(x|z)]}{E[\text{var}(y|z)]}.$$

This of course has the same drawback as the previous one if the variances are not independent of z.

Again assuming a model such as (10.1), we have that

$$\tau = \frac{E[\text{var}(x|z)]}{E[\text{var}(y|z)]} = \frac{\text{var}(x|z)}{\text{var}(y|z)} = \frac{\text{var}(y_{1ir})}{\text{var}(y_{2ir})} = \frac{\tau_1^2 + \sigma_1^2}{\tau_2^2 + \sigma_2^2}.$$

If we assume different replicates (i.e. comparing $\text{var}(y_{1ir})$ and $\text{var}(y_{2is})$), we get an extra term $2\omega^2$ in both numerator and denominator.

So τ is merely a comparison of the total variances of the two methods, which may be relevant or not, depending on the context. Whether it adds anything to the reporting of each of the variance components separately is doubtful, but the name of the index is indeed catchy.

10.4   Total deviation index

This measure was coined by Lin [19] as the value $\text{TDI}_{1-p} = \kappa$ such that a given fraction $(1 - p)$ of the differences between two methods will be in a symmetric interval $[-\kappa, \kappa]$. So, bar the uncertainty in the estimation of mean difference and the standard deviation of the differences, this is roughly equivalent to the numerically largest of the $1 - p$ limits of agreement.

The measure clearly has its main applicability in equivalence testing, where the interest is in establishing that a new drug or formulation deviates less than some prespecified number for a certain fraction of the patients (items in our terminology).

Lin [19] gives approximate formulae for the calculation of the measure, but it is a measure that easily lends itself to numerical calculation; one simply has to find TDI from the equation (assuming normality of the differences)

$$\Phi\left(\frac{\text{TDI} - \mu_d}{\sigma_d}\right) - \Phi\left(\frac{-\text{TDI} - \mu_d}{\sigma_d}\right) = 1 - p,$$

where μ_d and σ_d are the mean and standard deviation of the difference between measurements by method 1 and 2:

$$\mu_d = \alpha_1 - \alpha_2, \qquad \sigma_d = \sqrt{\tau_1^2 + \tau_2^2 + \sigma_1^2 + \sigma_2^2}.$$

If we want confidence limits for this, the simplest way to obtain them is by bootstrapping – in the case of a single measurement using resampling of data; in the case of a more complex model fitted with BUGS we may simply, for each posterior sample, plug in the values for μ_d and σ_d and solve for TDI.

What the measure adds to just taking the largest of the absolute values of the $(1 - p)$ limits of agreement is not really clear.

10.5   Correlation measures

The measures based on correlation are all by definition irrelevant in method comparison studies, because they involve the sample variation, i.e. the variation between items in the sample. This has repeatedly (and largely in vain) been pointed out in the literature [2, 3, 6]. However, I shall provide a summary of some of these measures in order to clarify how they relate to the parameters of the models we use.

Calculation of (some of) these measures is implemented in the `corr.measures()` function in the `MethComp` package, and there is a demonstration of their undesirable behavior in the example in the help file for the function.

The following is a brief overview in the context of the general model (7.1) introduced in Chapter 7 (omitting the method×replicate effect):

$$y_{mir} = \alpha_m + \beta_m \left(\mu_i + a_{ir} + c_{mi} \right) + e_{mir}.$$

However, in order to discuss the correlation measures proposed in the literature, we must modify the model by replacing the fixed item effects μ_i by random effects A_i, with variance ζ^2:

$$y_{mir} = \alpha_m + \beta_m \left(A_i + a_{ir} + c_{mi} \right) + e_{mir},$$

$$A_i \sim \mathcal{N}(0, \zeta^2), \quad a_{ir} \sim \mathcal{N}(0, \omega^2), \quad c_{mi} \sim \mathcal{N}(0, \tau_m^2),$$

$$e_{mir} \sim \mathcal{N}(0, \sigma_m^2).$$

(10.2)

This modification of the model is what it is all about; ζ is the standard deviation in the sample of items, and as such irrelevant for the comparison of methods. In any particular setting quite a wide range of ζ will be adequate for determination of the other parameters in the model. As will be clear from the next few sections, all measures proposed have the form

$$\frac{\zeta^2 + K_1}{\zeta^2 + K_2},$$

where K_1 and K_2 are functions of the other parameters in the model. So these measures all have the property that as the variation between items increases, so does the measure – even if the actual relationship between the methods is the same. This is why these measures are irrelevant; they mix the selection of items in where it does not belong.

10.5.1   Correlation coefficient

This measure is used mainly in a situation where we have one measurement by each method on each item, i.e. with no replicates. Under model (10.2) we have

$$\text{corr}(y_{1i}, y_{2i}) = \frac{\beta_1 \beta_2 (\zeta^2 + \omega^2)}{\sqrt{(\zeta^2 + \beta_1^2 \omega^2 + \beta_1^2 \tau_1^2 + \sigma_1^2)(\zeta^2 + \beta_2^2 \omega^2 + \beta_2^2 \tau_2^2 + \sigma_2^2)}}.$$

However, in the situation with only one measurement by each method, we cannot identify separate variances, the method×item (τ_m^2) interaction cannot be identified, and the item×replicate effect (ω^2) cannot be estimated because no replicates are available. Hence, we may just assume that $\omega = \tau_1 = \tau_2 = 0$ and that $\sigma_1 = \sigma_2$. This leads to the formula

$$\text{corr}(y_{1i}, y_{2i}) = \frac{\zeta^2}{\zeta^2 + \sigma^2}.$$

From this it is immediately clear that we are just looking at the ratio of the variation between items relative to the measurement variation. But since the variation between items is largely a quantity determined by the study design, we can pretty much get any value for the correlation by choosing the design accordingly – irrespective of the actual relationship between the *methods* of measurement.

10.5.2   Intraclass correlation coefficient

The intraclass correlation coefficient (ICC) is not a well-defined quantity in method comparison studies; basically there are two different scenarios, with and without replicate measurements.

In general, the ICC is defined in the framework of a one-way ANOVA with random group effect, i.e. a model

$$y_{ij} = \mu + A_i + e_{ij}, \qquad \text{var}(a_i) = \zeta^2, \quad \text{var}(e_{ij}) = \sigma^2,$$

and the ICC is defined as the correlation of two observations from the same group (= 'class'):

$$\text{ICC} = \text{corr}(y_{ij}, y_{ij'}) = \frac{\zeta^2}{\zeta^2 + \sigma^2}.$$

Single measurements

In the case of single measurements by each method, items are taken as groups and the measurements by each method as the replicates within each group. Note that is this case, measurements on the same item by different methods are considered exchangeable.

In terms of the model (10.2) this version of the ICC is not defined. Because of the exchangeability assumption we are operating in a model

$$y_{mi} = \mu + A_i + e_{mi}, \qquad A_i \sim \mathcal{N}(0, \zeta^2), \quad e_{mi} \sim \mathcal{N}(0, \sigma_m^2),$$

i.e. where the difference between the two methods a priori is assumed to be 0. In this setting, the ICC is $\zeta^2 / \sqrt{(\zeta^2 + \sigma_1^2)(\zeta^2 + \sigma_2^2)}$, which is equal to $\zeta^2 / (\zeta^2 + \sigma^2)$ if $\sigma_1 = \sigma_2$.

One way of computing this measure is to take a random half of the data points (y_{1i}, y_{2i}) and replace them by (y_{2i}, y_{1i}) (i.e. move the points to the other side of the identity line) and then compute the empirical correlation between y_1 and y_2. In order to get the right value one would of course have to do this repeatedly and average over the results.

But still ICC is comparing a measure of method precision (σ) to the variation between items (ζ).

Replicate measurements

In the case of replicate measurements it is possible to calculate the ICC separately for each method, by taking items as groups and using replicate measurements by the same method as replicates in each group.

In this case the residual variance component σ^2 measures the deviation for a given method from the method average for each item.

In terms of the model (10.2) this version of the ICC becomes

$$\text{ICC}_m = \frac{\beta_m^2(\zeta^2 + \tau_m^2)}{\beta_m^2(\zeta^2 + \omega^2 + \tau_m^2) + \sigma_m^2}, \tag{10.3}$$

or in the case of exchangeable replicates,

$$\text{ICC}_m = \frac{\beta_m^2(\zeta^2 + \tau_m^2)}{\beta_m^2(\zeta^2 + \tau_m^2) + \sigma_m^2}. \tag{10.4}$$

Again, we are relating a residual variance which is relevant for the evaluation of either the difference between methods or the repeatability of one method to the variation between items – the larger ζ, the larger the ICC.

Since the ICC_m is a measure of the precision for a single method it can be used to compare the precision between methods, because the irrelevant component, ζ^2, is the same for all methods – the method with the higher ICC has the better reproducibility. But a quick glance at formula (10.3) reveals that this can also be obtained more directly by comparing the variance components τ and σ between methods, so it is hard to see in this case what the ICC adds that is new.

10.5.3   Concordance correlation coefficient

Lin [18] proposed the concordance correlation coefficient (CCC) given by

$$\text{CCC} = 1 - \frac{\text{E}(y_{1i} - y_{2i})^2}{\text{var}(y_{1i}) + \text{var}(y_{2i}) + (\text{E}(y_{1i}) - \text{E}(y_{2i}))^2}.$$

The denominator is the expected value of the numerator under the assumption that measurements by method 1 and 2 are independent (i.e. totally unrelated). This is in itself quite a peculiar comparison basis, given that method comparison would expect from the outset that methods were measuring largely the same thing.

The CCC is thus a measure of the degree to which the correlation between the two methods of measurement changes the mean squared difference between the methods.

Under model (10.2) the numerator above is

$$E\left((\alpha_1 - \alpha_2 + (\beta_1 - \beta_2)(A_i + a_{ir}) + \beta_1 c_{1i} - \beta_2 c_{2i} + e_{1ir} - e_{2ir})^2\right)$$

$$= (\alpha_1 - \alpha_2)^2 + (\beta_1 - \beta_2)^2(\zeta^2 + \omega^2) + \beta_1^2\tau_1^2 + \beta_2^2\tau_2^2 + \sigma_1^2 + \sigma_2^2$$

because all the random effects are assumed independent. The denominator is

$$(\beta_1^2 + \beta_2^2)(\zeta^2 + \omega^2) + \beta_1^2\tau_1^2 + \beta_2^2\tau_2^2 + \sigma_1^2 + \sigma_2^2 + (\alpha_1 - \alpha_2)^2.$$

Therefore under the model the CCC is

$$CCC = \frac{2\beta_1\beta_2(\zeta^2 + \omega^2)}{(\alpha_1 - \alpha_2)^2 + (\beta_1^2 + \beta_2^2)(\zeta^2 + \omega^2) + \beta_1^2\tau_1^2 + \beta_2^2\tau_2^2 + \sigma_1^2 + \sigma_2^2}.$$

If we are in the situation with one measurement per item on each of two methods, we cannot identify ω and we cannot have separate estimates of τ and σ, so the expression becomes

$$CCC = \frac{2\beta_1\beta_2\zeta^2}{(\alpha_1 + \alpha_2)^2 + (\beta_1^2 + \beta_2^2)\zeta^2 + 2\sigma^2}.$$

If we further assume that the bias between the methods is constant we have $\beta_1 = \beta_2 = 1$, leading to

$$CCC = \frac{2\zeta^2}{(\alpha_1 + \alpha_2)^2 + 2\zeta^2 + 2\sigma^2}.$$

In any case it is clear that the CCC is a measure that increases toward 1 as the variation between items (ζ^2) increases. This was pointed out shortly after the publication of Lin's paper [18] by Atkinson and Nevill [3].

10.6 Summary

As we have seen, various summary measures are either ratios of subsets of the variance components or, if these are not constant over the range of measurements, weighted averages of these using the empirical distribution of measurements as weights. In the first case the added value is small, in the latter case almost certainly non-existent but definitely irrelevant.

Barnhart *et al.* in their review [4] state that: 'The ICC, CCC and DC are related and depend on between-subject variability and may produce high values for heterogeneous populations [3, 8]'. This statement is as clear as any in dismissing these measures as being irrelevant for clinical method comparison studies: no one would want a measure that depends on the particular sample used for the comparison. Nor would anyone want to refer to a 'population' in the context of a method comparison study.

Of the measures mentioned in this section only the IBC has an immediate (relevant) interpretability.

11

Design of method comparison studies

Two aspects of designing studies of method comparisons are of primary concern:

1. The choice of items to analyze, i.e. the number and the spread of the true values. The latter is of course not known a priori but usually some handle on these values can be obtained from persons handling the measurements in daily practice. In practical situations it will involve choosing items (persons) with and without disease, or in different age ranges, etc.

2. The experimental design, i.e.:

   • how many item should be included;

   • how many replicates by each method;

   • how and when replicates are made.

   Only the two first questions here lend themselves to general recommendations, the last being necessarily context-specific.

Comparing Clinical Measurement Methods: A Practical Guide   Bendix Carstensen
© 2010 John Wiley & Sons, Ltd

11.1   Sample size

There are two sets of parameters of interest in a method comparison study: the mean parameters, governing the relationship between the means of measurements; and the variance parameters, describing the uncertainty within and between the methods. To the extent that we have a reasonable handle on the mean and variance parameters, we can simulate data from an experiment, analyze the simulated data and get a feeling for the precision of the estimates. Traditional power calculations are irrelevant in method comparisons, because the endeavor inherently is about estimation and not about hypothesis testing.

11.1.1   Mean parameters

The mean parameters are not of interest *per se*; it is the precision of the mean conversion equations between methods that is of interest. In practice it is difficult to say anything sensible about the sample size needed for a given precision, because it depends both on the variances and the layout. Basically the only general advice that can be given is to choose the items used in the study as evenly spread as possible over the clinically relevant range.

11.1.2   Variance parameters

In general quite a lot of observations are required to produce stable variance estimates. This means that the limiting factor in study design is the estimation of the variance components; the mean difference and the slope linking methods will be sufficiently precisely determined if the variance components are.

Under the simplest possible assumptions about the distributions of variance estimates, these follow a scaled χ^2 distribution. This means that a confidence interval (c.i.) for an estimate of a variance (on f degrees of freedom (d.f.)) is obtained by multiplying the estimated value by $f/\chi^2_{0.975}(f)$ and by $f/\chi^2_{0.025}(f)$. Since we are interested the precision of the standard deviations of the random effects in the models, we need the square root of these factors:

| d.f. | c.i. multiplier | | d.f. | c.i. multiplier | |
	lower	upper		lower	upper
20	0.77	1.44	100	0.88	1.16
30	0.80	1.34	150	0.90	1.13
40	0.82	1.28	200	0.91	1.11
42	0.82	1.27	250	0.92	1.10
50	0.84	1.24	300	0.93	1.09
60	0.85	1.22	350	0.93	1.08
70	0.86	1.20	400	0.94	1.07
80	0.87	1.18	450	0.94	1.07
90	0.87	1.17	500	0.94	1.07

From the table it is evident that there is not much to gain in terms of precision beyond 40 or 50 degrees of freedom unless massive studies are to be set up, so a bold recommendation in terms of d.f. for variance estimates would be 42.[1]

This would give confidence intervals for the standard deviations which, broadly speaking, are constructed by multiplying and dividing the estimate by 1.25, and so in most practical situations would still be the dominating source of uncertainty in the resulting conversion equations.

Thus the central quantity to regulate is the number of degrees of freedom underlying the variance estimates. The variance components of primary interest are the method×item and the residual variance. The random item×replicate interaction included with linked replicates has more the character of a nuisance parameter which we must include in the model to get the other variances estimated correctly.

From the approximate analysis of variance diagram (7.3) shown on page 70, we can see that the approximate degrees of freedom for the method×item effects are $(M - 1)(I - 2)$, so to attain 42 d.f. by two methods the recommendation would be 44 items, but for $M = 3$ we need to estimate three variances, i.e. we would recommend $2(I - 1) = 126 \Rightarrow I = 64$ items.

---

[1] See Douglas Adams, *The Hitch-hiker's Guide to the Galaxy*, in which Deep Thought computed the Answer to the Ultimate Question of Life, the Universe, and Everything as 42.

From the same display we see that the degrees of freedom for the residual variation are $I\left((M-1)(R-1)-1\right)$, so for two methods with 44 items, we would need four replicates per method×item to achieve $44\left((2-1)(4-1)-1\right)) = 88$ d.f., i.e. 44 d.f. for each of the two variances. For three methods we could get away with three replicates per method if we include 64 items: $64\left((3-1)(3-1)-1\right)) = 192$ d.f., i.e. 64 d.f. per variance.

So in broad terms the recommendation would be around 50 items with three replicate measurements on each method.

So far we have assumed that the design was completely described by method, item and replicate, i.e. a subset of a complete three-way layout, possibly without replicates (which would be a two-way layout).

11.2   Repeated measures designs

A common design is one where repeated measures are taken on the same persons, e.g. blood samples may be taken at different times during some experiment, and all samples are analyzed by two or more methods. In this case it is not clear whether the blood sample or the person should be regarded as the item.

If we regard the blood sample as the item, we do not have replicate measurements by each method, so method-specific variability cannot be estimated. However, we may impose assumptions on the sources of variation that allow us to do so anyway. Assume that data are classified by method (m), person (p) and time (t). Assuming that the blood sample plays the role of the item ($i = (p, t)$), we would use a model

$$y_{mpt} = \alpha_m + \beta_m \mu_{pt} + e_{mpt}.$$

In this setup we actually do have the possibility of splitting the error term and estimating a method×person effect. The method×person effect would be interpreted as a matrix effect, i.e. a person-specific deviation common to all methods used to analyze samples from that person and entered in the model as a random effect, thus the model specification would be

$$y_{mpt} = \alpha_m + \beta_m \mu_{pt} + c_{mp} + e_{mpt},$$

$$c_{mp} \sim \mathcal{N}(0, \tau_m^2) e_{mpt} \sim \mathcal{N}(0, \sigma_m^2).$$

This is the same model as we arrived at when discussing changing the random item×replicate effect to a fixed effect, a model without replicates.

Therefore, when we have a time dimension to the replicates it is recommended to include a random item×replicate (i.e. item×time) effect and, to the extent that we are interested in time trajectories, to include a systematic time effect in the model.

11.3   Summary

In most cases 50 items (persons, samples) with three replicate measurements by each method will provide reasonable precision for the parameters of interest, both the mean relation between methods and the variance components. The latter will be determined with an uncertainty of about 25% on either side.

12

Examples using
standard software

As far as estimation goes, the standard software only covers the situation with constant bias, so this is what is covered in this chapter. The next chapter contains a brief introduction to the `MethComp` package for R, which has functions that also handle non-constant bias.

In this chapter it is assumed that the data is in a data set given in the 'long' form, i.e. with one measurement per line, and that the data set has variables called `meth`, `item`, `repl` and `y`, the latter being the measurements.

To illustrate the case with exchangeable replicates we will use the fat data from Section 2.2.1 above, and for the case of linked replicates we will use both the data on cardiac output from Table 4 and the data on systolic blood pressure measurement from Table 1, both in [8]. The data sets are available on-line so that you can try out the code.

The example data sets are available as follows:

fat, `http://staff.pubhealth.ku.dk/~bxc/MethComp/` `Book/Data/fat.txt`;

cardiac, `http://staff.pubhealth.ku.dk/~bxc/MethComp/` `Book/Data/cardiac.txt`;

systolic blood pressure, `http://staff.pubhealth.ku.dk/` `~bxc/MethComp/Book/Data/sbp.txt`.

Comparing Clinical Measurement Methods: A Practical Guide   Bendix Carstensen
© 2010 John Wiley & Sons, Ltd

All three data sets have been converted to long form and have a first line with the variable names.

The systolic blood pressure example is not analyzed in Stata or SAS, because both programs crash when fitting the model for these data (it has three methods, linked replicates and separate method×item variance for each method).

All the programs used can be found in the folder http://staff. pubhealth.ku.dk/~bxc/MethComp/Book/Programs, so that you should be able to reproduce the analyses shown here by yourself.

12.1 SAS

12.1.1 Exchangeable replicates

We use the fat data to illustrate the SAS code needed to produce the results.

```
filename fatfile url
  "http://staff.pubhealth.ku.dk/~bxc/MethComp/Book/Data/fat.txt" ;

data fat ;
  infile fatfile firstobs=2 ;
  input meth $ item repl y ;
run ;
```

```
NOTE: 258 records were read from the infile FATFILE.
      The minimum record length was 8.
      The maximum record length was 12.
NOTE: The data set WORK.FAT has 258 observations and 4 variables.
NOTE: DATA statement used (Total process time):
      real time          0.26 seconds
      cpu time           0.00 seconds
```

We need to declare meth and item as class variables for proc mixed to recognize them as such. In order to get method-specific residual variances estimated we need a repeated statement with /group=meth:

```
proc mixed  data = fat ;
  class meth item ;
  model y = meth item / s;
  random meth * item ;
  repeated / group = meth ;
run ;
```

```
NOTE: Convergence criteria met.
```

```
NOTE: The PROCEDURE MIXED printed pages 1-2.
NOTE: PROCEDURE MIXED used (Total process time):
      real time          3.24 seconds
      cpu time           1.09 seconds

Number of Observations Read            258
Number of Observations Used            258
Number of Observations Not Used          0

Iteration History
Iteration    Evaluations    -2 Res Log Like       Criterion
        0              1       -353.24387418
        1              1       -376.69765836      0.00000000
Convergence criteria met.

Covariance Parameter Estimates
Cov Parm        Group       Estimate
meth*item                   0.003547
Residual       meth KL      0.005956
Residual       meth SL      0.005244

Solution for Fixed Effects
                                          Standard
Effect      meth    item    Estimate       Error     DF    t Value    Pr > |t|
Intercept                     1.6277      0.05259     42      30.95     <.0001
meth        KL                0.04488     0.01587     42       2.83     0.0071
meth        SL                0             .          .        .         .
item                1         0.01703     0.07356     42       0.23     0.8180
item                2        -0.8483      0.07356     42     -11.53     <.0001
item                3         1.1496      0.07356     42      15.63     <.0001
item                4        -0.9908      0.07356     42     -13.47     <.0001
item                5         1.2185      0.07356     42      16.56     <.0001
...
```

From the output we find that the estimated difference under the fixed effect is 0.04488, meaning that the observer KL measures on average 0.045 mm more than SL.

The estimate of the *variance* of the method×item effect is 0.003547, so the standard deviation is $\sqrt{0.003547} = 0.05956$, identical for the two methods, and the estimated residual variances are 0.005956 for KL and 0.005244 for SL, so the standard deviations are 0.07718 and 0.07242, respectively.

These are the quantities needed to report the simple model with constant bias, and the limits of agreement for KL−SL are thus

$$0.04488 \pm 2 \times \sqrt{2 \times 0.003547 + 0.005244 + 0.005956}$$
$$= 0.045 \pm 0.271 = (-0.226, 0.315).$$

12.1.2   Linked replicates

In this section we use the cardiac data to show how to accommodate
linked replicates when comparing two methods (the `cardiac` data,
comparing methods IC and RV).

```
filename cardfile url
  "http://staff.pubhealth.ku.dk/~bxc/MethComp/Data/Book/cardiac.txt" ;

data cardiac ;
  infile cardfile firstobs=2 ;
  input meth $ item repl y ;
run ;
```

```
NOTE: 120 records were read from the infile CARDFILE.
      The minimum record length was 9.
      The maximum record length was 12.
NOTE: The data set WORK.CARDIAC has 120 observations and 4 variables.
NOTE: DATA statement used (Total process time):
      real time        1.06 seconds
      cpu time         0.00 seconds
```

In order to fit the model for linked replicates we must include the
item×replicate interaction as a random effect:

```
proc mixed  data = cardiac ;
  class meth item repl ;
  model y = meth item / s;
  random meth*item  item*repl ;
  repeated / group=meth ;
run ;
```

```
Number of Observations Read            120
Number of Observations Used            120
Number of Observations Not Used          0
```

```
Iteration History
Iteration     Evaluations     -2 Res Log Like      Criterion
        0               1        214.58537627
        1               2        137.19341656      0.02692572
        2               2        136.26965851      0.00218142
        3               1        136.19985796      0.00002067
        4               1        136.19922909      0.00000000
Convergence criteria met.
```

```
Covariance Parameter Estimates
Cov Parm      Group        Estimate
meth*item                   0.4364
item*repl                   0.03717
Residual      meth IC       0.1007
Residual      meth RV       0.07007
```

```
Solution for Fixed Effects
```

Effect	meth	item	Estimate	Standard Error	DF	t Value	Pr > |t|
Intercept			4.8924	0.5002	11	9.78	<.0001
meth	IC		-0.7045	0.2752	11	-2.56	0.0265
meth	RV		0	.	.	.	.
item		1	2.4766	0.6824	11	3.63	0.0040
item		2	0.8886	0.6853	11	1.30	0.2213
item		3	0.7150	0.6805	11	1.05	0.3159
item		4	-0.3448	0.6824	11	-0.51	0.6234
item		5	-1.6901	0.6805	11	-2.48	0.0304
item		6	1.4209	0.6853	11	2.07	0.0624
item		7	1.3001	0.6853	11	1.90	0.0844
item		8	0.2232	0.6805	11	0.33	0.7490
item		9	-0.7664	0.6901	11	-1.11	0.2904
item		10	-0.3662	0.6824	11	-0.54	0.6022
item		11	2.0853	0.6805	11	3.06	0.0108
item		12	0	.	.	.	.

From the output we see that the mean difference between the methods is -0.7045, the variance of the method×item effects is 0.4364 and the residual variances are 0.1007 and 0.07007, respectively. This corresponds to standard deviations of the effects of 0.661, 0.317 and 0.265, respectively.

The item×replicate variance is 0.03717, i.e. the standard deviation is 0.193, but recall that this figure is not related to the issue of method comparison, but more to the design of the study.

The limits of agreement for IC−RV are therefore

$$-0.7045 \pm 2 \times \sqrt{2 \times 0.4364 + 0.1007 + 0.07007}$$

$$= -0.70 \pm 2.04 = (-2.75, 1.34).$$

12.2   Stata

12.2.1   Exchangeable replicates

We use the fat data to illustrate the required Stata code needed for this analysis.

```
. insheet using "http://staff.pubhealth.ku.dk/~bxc/MethComp/Data/fat.txt",
clear names delim(" ")
```

```
(4 vars, 258 obs)
```

We need to declare an explicit numerical indicator variable for one of the methods (the one with the larger residual variance) in order to be able to specify a model with method-specific residual variances.

Moreover, we need to specify the interactions we need, explicitly in order to get them into `xtmixed`:

```
. gen meth1 = ( meth == "KL" )
. gen MI = item + 100 * meth1
. gen MIR = _n
.
. xi: xtmixed y i.meth1 i.item  || MI: || MIR:meth1, nocons var

i.meth1          _Imeth1_0-1        (naturally coded; _Imeth1_0 omitted)
i.item           _Iitem_1-46        (naturally coded; _Iitem_1 omitted)

Performing EM optimization:
Performing gradient-based optimization:
Iteration 0:  log restricted-likelihood =   185.333
Iteration 1:  log restricted-likelihood = 188.27598
Iteration 2:  log restricted-likelihood = 188.34852
Iteration 3:  log restricted-likelihood = 188.34884
Iteration 4:  log restricted-likelihood = 188.34884

Computing standard errors:
Mixed-effects REML regression          Number of obs = 258
------------------------------------------------------------
                  | No. of     Observations per Group
 Group Variable |  Groups   Minimum   Average   Maximum
----------------+-------------------------------------------
           MI |     86         3        3.0        3
          MIR |    258         1        1.0        1
------------------------------------------------------------
                         Wald chi2(43) = 11799.40
Log restricted-likelihood = 188.34884  Prob > chi2  =   0.0000
------------------------------------------------------------------------
       y |   Coef.    Std. Err.     z    P>|z|   [95% Conf. Interval]
---------+--------------------------------------------------------------
_Imeth1_1 |  .0448837  .015868    2.83   0.005   .0137829   .0759845
_Iitem_2 | -.8653287  .0735594  -11.76   0.000  -1.009502  -.7211549
_Iitem_3 |  1.132603  .0735594   15.40   0.000   .9884293   1.276777
_Iitem_4 | -1.007786  .0735594  -13.70   0.000  -1.151959  -.8636119
_Iitem_5 |  1.201461  .0735594   16.33   0.000   1.057287   1.345634
_Iitem_6 | -.7673239  .0735594  -10.43   0.000  -.9114977  -.6231502
...
_Iitem_46 | -.0170318  .0735594   -0.23   0.817  -.1612056   .1271419
    _cons |  1.644717  .05259     31.27   0.000   1.541642   1.747791
------------------------------------------------------------------------


------------------------------------------------------------------------
 Random-effects Parameters |  Estimate   Std. Err.   [95% Conf. Interval]
---------------------------+--------------------------------------------
MI: Identity    var(_cons) |  .0035469  .0011984   .0018291   .0068779
---------------------------+--------------------------------------------
MIR: Identity   var(meth1) |  .0007116  .0012102   .0000254   .0199439
---------------------------+--------------------------------------------
```

```
            var(Residual) |    .0052442    .0007997      .0038893    .0070711
-----------------------------------------------------------------------------
LR test vs. linear regression:        chi2(2) =    23.45   Prob > chi2 = 0.0000

Note: LR test is conservative and provided only for reference.
```

From the output we find an estimated difference under the fixed effect of 0.0448837 (_Imeth1_1), meaning that the observer KL measures on average 0.045 cm more than KL.

The estimate of the *variance* of the method×item effect is 0.0035469, so the standard deviation is $\sqrt{0.0035469} = 0.0596$, identical for the two methods. Stata parametrizes by the *difference* between the variances, so the estimated residual variances are 0.0052442 for SL and $0.0052442 + 0.0007116 = 0.0059558$ for KL (because the meth1 variable was defined as the indicator of KL); that is, the standard deviations are 0.0772 and 0.0724, respectively.

These are the quantities needed to report the simple model with constant bias; the limits of agreement for KL−SL will be

$$0.044 \pm 2 \times \sqrt{2 \times 0.0035469 + 0.0052442 + 0.0059558}$$
$$= 0.044 \pm 0.271 = (-0.227, 0.315).$$

12.2.2 Linked replicates

In this section we use the cardiac data to show how to accommodate linked replicates when comparing two methods.

As previously, we need to generate numerical indicators of the methods, and variables with the desired interactions:

```
. insheet using "http://staff.pubhealth.ku.dk/~bxc/MethComp/Data/cardiac.txt",
clear names delim(" ")

(4 vars, 120 obs)

. gen meth1 = (meth=="IC")
. gen meth2 = (meth=="RV")
. gen MI = item + 100 * meth1
. gen IR = item + 100 * repl
. gen MIR = _n
```

In order to fit the model for linked replicates we must include the item×replicate interaction as a random effect:

```
. xi:xtmixed y i.meth i.item || _all:R.MI || _all:R.IR || MIR:meth1, nocons var

i.meth          _Imeth_1-2         (_Imeth_1 for meth==IC omitted)
i.item          _Iitem_1-12        (naturally coded; _Iitem_1 omitted)

Performing EM optimization:
Performing gradient-based optimization:
Iteration 0:    log restricted-likelihood = -71.174897   (not concave)
Iteration 1:    log restricted-likelihood = -68.144061
Iteration 2:    log restricted-likelihood = -68.101706
Iteration 3:    log restricted-likelihood = -68.099626
Iteration 4:    log restricted-likelihood = -68.09962

Computing standard errors:
Mixed-effects REML regression                   Number of obs      =      120
-----------------------------------------------------------------
                |   No. of        Observations per Group
Group Variable  |   Groups    Minimum    Average    Maximum
----------------+------------------------------------------------
          _all  |      1        120       120.0        120
           MIR  |    120          1         1.0          1
-----------------------------------------------------------------


                                         Wald chi2(12)      =     76.11
Log restricted-likelihood = -68.09962    Prob > chi2        =    0.0000
------------------------------------------------------------------------------
        y  |    Coef.    Std. Err.      z     P>|z|    [95% Conf. Interval]
----------+-------------------------------------------------------------------
 _Imeth_2 |   .704521   .2751588      2.56    0.010    .1652197    1.243822
 _Iitem_2 | -1.588028    .687255     -2.31    0.021   -2.935023   -.2410325
 _Iitem_3 | -1.761681   .6824017     -2.58    0.010   -3.099164   -.4241981
 _Iitem_4 | -2.821403   .6843474     -4.12    0.000     -4.1627   -1.480107
 _Iitem_5 |  -4.16676   .6824017     -6.11    0.000   -5.504243   -2.829277
 _Iitem_6 | -1.055789    .687255     -1.54    0.124   -2.402784     .291206
 _Iitem_7 | -1.176507    .687255     -1.71    0.087   -2.523502    .1704882
 _Iitem_8 | -2.253414   .6824017     -3.30    0.001   -3.590897   -.9159313
 _Iitem_9 | -3.243087   .6920721     -4.69    0.000   -4.599523    -1.88665
_Iitem_10 | -2.842873   .6843474     -4.15    0.000   -4.184169   -1.501577
_Iitem_11 |  -.3913089  .6824017     -0.57    0.566   -1.728792    .9461739
_Iitem_12 | -2.476644   .6824017     -3.63    0.000   -3.814126   -1.139161
     _cons |  6.664502   .5033395     13.24    0.000    5.677975     7.65103
------------------------------------------------------------------------------


------------------------------------------------------------------------------
  Random-effects Parameters  |  Estimate   Std. Err.    [95% Conf. Interval]
-----------------------------+------------------------------------------------
_all: Identity    var(R.MI)  |  .4364029    .194185     .1824445    1.043865
-----------------------------+------------------------------------------------
_all: Identity    var(R.IR)  |  .0371726   .0183569     .0141213    .0978523
-----------------------------+------------------------------------------------
MIR: Identity    var(meth1)  |  .0306623   .0340158     .0034858    .2697133
-----------------------------+------------------------------------------------
               var(Residual) |   .07007    .0220057     .0378625    .1296747
------------------------------------------------------------------------------
LR test vs. linear regression:         chi2(3) =    78.39   Prob > chi2 = 0.0000
Note: LR test is conservative and provided only for reference.
```

From the output we see that the mean difference between the methods is 0.704521 (at `_Imeth_2`), the variance of the method×item effects is 0.4364029 and the residual variance in `meth2`, that is the RV group, is 0.07007 and that the difference between the residual variance in the IC and the RV groups is 0.0306623, i.e. that residual variance in the IC group is $0.07007 + 0.0306623 = 0.1007323$. This corresponds to standard deviations of the effects of 0.661, 0.317 and 0.265, respectively.

The item×replicate variance is 0.03717, i.e. the standard deviation is 0.193, but recall that this figure is not related to the issue of method comparison, but more to the design of the study.

The limits of agreement for IC−RV are therefore

$$-0.704521 \pm 2 \times \sqrt{2 \times 0.4364029 + 0.1007323 + 0.07007}$$

$$= -0.70 \pm 2.04 = (-2.75, 1.34).$$

12.3   R

The examples given here can be run more smoothly by using the functions from the `MethComp` package tailored for these kinds of analyses. The algorithms run are the same, but they are nicely wrapped. The `MethComp` package is treated in Chapter 13.

12.3.1   Exchangeable replicates

```
> fat <- read.table( url(
+ "http://staff.pubhealth.ku.dk/~bxc/MethComp/Book/Data/fat.txt"),
+                 header=TRUE )
> fat$meth <- factor( fat$meth )
> fat$item <- factor( fat$item )
> fat$repl <- factor( fat$repl )
> str( fat )

'data.frame': 258 obs. of  4 variables:
 $ meth: Factor w/ 2 levels "KL","SL": 1 1 1 1 1 1 1 1 1 1 ...
 $ item: Factor w/ 43 levels "1","2","3","4",..: 1 1 1 3 3 3 5 5 5 11 ...
 $ repl: Factor w/ 3 levels "1","2","3": 1 2 3 1 2 3 1 2 3 1 ...
 $ y   : num  1.6 1.7 1.7 2.8 2.9 2.8 2.7 2.8 2.9 3.9 ...
```

The convention in `lme` is that the name of the first element of the list in the `random` argument is the name of the variable within which the rest of the effects are nested. Hence we need to nest `meth` within `item` in order to get the method×item interaction.

```
> library( nlme )
> lme( y ~ meth + item,
+        random = list( item = pdIdent( ~ meth-1 ) ),
+        weights = varIdent( form = ~ 1 | meth ),
+        data=fat
+      )

Linear mixed-effects model fit by REML
  Data: fat
  Log-restricted-likelihood: 188.3488
  Fixed: y ~ meth + item
  (Intercept)        methSL        item2        item3        item4
   1.6896001995 -0.0448837209 -0.8653286307  1.1326030428 -1.0077856154
         item5        item6        item7        item8        item9
   1.2014605811 -0.7673239281 -0.1844287691 -0.2510954358  0.6155712309
        item10       item11       item13       item14       item15
  -0.5496348547  2.1282212996 -0.6750365145  1.2326030428 -0.9973239281
        item16       item17       item18       item19       item20
  -0.3851590597 -0.0007302905 -0.0844287691 -0.0836984786  0.1815076070
        item21       item22       item24       item25       item27
  -0.4347939144  0.2510954358  0.3170318119  0.0496348547 -0.4503651453
        item28       item29       item30       item31       item32
  -1.0365206086  0.9318727523  0.3163015214  0.0992697095 -1.1891236514
        item33       item34       item35       item36       item37
  -0.0333333333  2.1163015214  0.8170318119  0.3815076070  1.4666666667
        item38       item39       item40       item41       item42
  -0.4666666667 -0.7991236514  0.8518257263  2.4148409403 -0.4666666667
        item43       item44       item45       item46
  -0.1170318119  0.2496348547  0.1481742737 -0.0170318119

Random effects:
 Formula: ~meth - 1 | item
 Structure: Multiple of an Identity
           methKL    methSL   Residual
 StdDev: 0.059556 0.059556 0.07717392

Variance function:
 Structure: Different standard deviations per stratum
 Formula: ~1 | meth
 Parameter estimates:
        KL        SL
 1.0000000 0.9383578
Number of Observations: 258
Number of Groups: 43
```

From the output we find an estimated difference under the fixed effect of -0.0448837209, meaning that the observer SL measures on average 0.045 mm less than KL.

R parametrizes the residual as the standard deviation in one group, and the ratio of the standard deviations in the other groups relative to this.

The estimate of the method×item standard deviation is 0.059556, identical for the two methods, and the estimate of the residual standard deviation is 0.07717392 in the reference group (KL) and 0.07717392 × 0.9383578 = 0.07241675 in the other group.

These are the quantities needed to report the simple model with constant bias.

12.3.2 Linked replicates

In this section we show how to accommodate both the case with two methods (the cardiac data) and with three methods of measurement (the systolic blood pressure data).

Cardiac data

```
> card <- read.table( url(
+ "http://staff.pubhealth.ku.dk/~bxc/MethComp/Book/Data/cardiac.txt"),
+                 header=TRUE )
> card$meth <- factor( card$meth )
> card$item <- factor( card$item )
> card$repl <- factor( card$repl )
> str( card )

'data.frame': 120 obs. of  4 variables:
 $ meth: Factor w/ 2 levels "IC","RV": 2 2 2 2 2 2 2 2 2 2 ...
 $ item: Factor w/ 12 levels "1","2","3","4",..: 1 1 1 1 1 2 2 2 2 3 ...
 $ repl: Factor w/ 6 levels "1","2","3","4",..: 1 2 3 4 5 1 2 3 4 1 ...
 $ y   : num  7.83 7.42 7.89 7.12 7.88 6.16 7.26 6.71 6.54 4.75 ...
```

In order to fit the model for linked replicates we must include the item×replicate interaction, which is done by putting the term repl = 1 in the random list. The first element in the list is item, so the rest of the list is nested in this:

```
> lme( y ~ meth + item,
+          random = list( item = pdIdent( ~ meth-1 ),
+                         repl = ~ 1 ),
+          weights = varIdent( form = ~1 | meth ),
+          data = card
+          )

Linear mixed-effects model fit by REML
  Data: card
  Log-restricted-likelihood: -68.09961
  Fixed: y ~ meth + item
(Intercept)       methRV        item2        item3        item4        item5
  6.6645025    0.7045210   -1.5880276   -1.7616809   -2.8214031   -4.1667599
       item6        item7        item8        item9       item10       item11
```

```
-1.0557890  -1.1765069  -2.2534141  -3.2430868  -2.8428729  -0.3913089
    item12
-2.4766435

Random effects:
 Formula: ~meth - 1 | item
 Structure: Multiple of an Identity
         methIC    methRV
StdDev: 0.6606085 0.6606085

 Formula: ~1 | repl %in% item
       (Intercept)   Residual
StdDev:   0.192802 0.2647074

Variance function:
 Structure: Different standard deviations per stratum
 Formula: ~1 | meth
 Parameter estimates:
      RV        IC
1.000000 1.198997
Number of Observations: 120
Number of Groups:
        item repl %in% item
          12            60
```

Note that in this model we have assumed that the size of the method×item is the same for both methods (the `pdIdent` function), as this is the only possibility with two methods.

From the output we see that the mean difference between the methods is 0.7045, the standard deviation of the method×item effect is 0.6606 and the residual standard deviations are 0.2647 and 0.2647074 × 1.198997 = 0.3174, respectively. The item×replicate standard deviation is 0.1928, but recall that this figure is not related to the method comparison, but only to the study design.

Blood pressure data

This example illustrates the case of linked replicates in the situation with three methods, where it is possible to estimate method-specific variances of the method×item effects.

```
> sbp <- read.table( url(
+ "http://staff.pubhealth.ku.dk/~bxc/MethComp/Book/Data/sbp.txt"),
+                     header=TRUE )
> sbp$meth <- factor( sbp$meth )
> sbp$item <- factor( sbp$item )
> sbp$repl <- factor( sbp$repl )
> str( sbp )
```

```
'data.frame': 765 obs. of  4 variables:
$ meth: Factor w/ 3 levels "J","R","S": 1 1 1 1 1 1 1 1 1 1 ...
$ item: Factor w/ 85 levels "1","2","3","4",..: 1 2 3 4 5 6 7 8 9 10 ...
$ repl: Factor w/ 3 levels "1","2","3": 1 1 1 1 1 1 1 1 1 1 ...
$ y   : int  100 108 76 108 124 122 116 114 100 108 ...
```

In order to fit the model for linked replicates we must include the item×replicate interaction:

```
> lme( y ~ meth + item,
+           random = list( item = pdIdent( ~ meth-1 ),
+                          repl = ~ 1 ),
+           weights = varIdent( form = ~1 | meth ),
+           data = sbp
+           )
```

This specifies a model where we assume that the size of the method×item is the same for all three methods (output not shown). In order to get method-specific values for the method×item effect, we must use pdDiag instead of pdIdent in the specification of the effect:

```
> lme( y ~ meth + item,
+           random = list( item = pdDiag( ~ meth-1 ),
+                          repl = ~ 1 ),
+           weights = varIdent( form = ~1 | meth ),
+           data = sbp
+           )

Linear mixed-effects model fit by REML
  Data: sbp
  Log-restricted-likelihood: -2197.298
  Fixed: y ~meth + item
  (Intercept)        methR        methS        item2        item3        item4
 103.27571236  -0.08627451  15.61960784   6.18117844 -21.82090409   2.11645404
        item5        item6        item7        item8        item9       item10
  13.88374759  26.17326485   6.16868331   8.03590248   3.06680692  -2.11500290
       item11       item12       item13       item14       item15       item16
   1.20625181  11.13611286   8.47652676   2.10562493   1.36840281  15.36756980
       item17       item18       item19       item20       item21       item22
  -1.90103914  14.67258084  33.33133392  43.34049702  53.28868426  39.79174878
       item23       item24       item25       item26       item27       item28
  65.93119367  60.82493736  39.43437671  27.43271070  37.72930854  45.40563791
       item29       item30       item31       item32       item33       item34
 116.09604533  95.62335021 -14.85847259  15.13652936  18.68257694  21.93744124
       item35       item36       item37       item38       item39       item40
  16.08688223 -12.64950688   4.47402774 105.34299604  24.98792137  30.76604403
       item41       item42       item43       item44       item45       item46
  -8.93527561  -7.90353817  17.79903098  58.77562363  -1.82215360  24.40680432
       item47       item48       item49       item50       item51       item52
  11.45062038  31.63463124  49.40938645 -11.50722957  52.69757110  -1.23145694
       item53       item54       item55       item56       item57       item58
   1.51950982  -4.18139331 -23.80007887   1.73805513   5.87500099  75.88374759
       item59       item60       item61       item62       item63       item64
  53.05639431  36.04006753  93.80861058 -11.62151798  24.41013635  37.06347488
```

```
      item65         item66         item67         item68         item69         item70
 33.73763863   54.19742211   29.74638522    9.88149885   13.44062428   17.80361253
      item71         item72         item73         item74         item75         item76
112.67841190   30.81977309   54.08729874  -19.24020353   70.83534997   75.73972115
      item77         item78         item79         item80         item81         item82
 13.47186211   15.47627744    4.77853916    6.49676926   37.19542269    5.23415760
      item83         item84         item85
  7.05972634   -1.87146733   12.83784900

Random effects:
 Formula: ~meth - 1 | item
 Structure: Diagonal
            methJ         methR     methS
 StdDev: 0.3384723 0.001055065 18.07713

 Formula: ~1 | repl %in% item
         (Intercept) Residual
 StdDev:    5.887152 1.630053

Variance function:
 Structure: Different standard deviations per stratum
 Formula: ~1 | meth
 Parameter estimates:
         J         R         S
 1.0000000 0.9488457 5.6089019
Number of Observations: 765
Number of Groups:
         item repl %in% item
           85             255
```

Then we have the possibility of fishing out the relevant estimates for these three methods; the mean estimates, i.e. average differences with respect to the reference method J, are -0.08627451 and 15.61960784 for methods R and S, respectively. The method×item standard deviations are 0.3384723, 0.001055065 and 18.07713.

The residual standard deviation is given as 1.630053 in the reference group, and the multipliers that give us the residual standard deviation in each of the groups are 1.0000000, 0.9488457 and 5.6089019, giving residual standard deviations of

$$1.630053 \times (1.0000000, 0.9488457, 5.6089019)$$
$$= (1.630053, 1.546669, 9.142807).$$

The item×replicate standard deviation is 5.887152; however, this is not an effect of any predictive relevance. But it indicates that the variation between replicates is rather large; omitting this gives dramatically larger residual standard deviations:

```
> lme( y ~ meth + item,
+          random = list( item = pdDiag( ~ meth-1 ) ),
+          weights = varIdent( form = ~ 1 | meth ),
+          data = sbp
+     )
```

```
Linear mixed-effects model fit by REML
 Data: sbp
 Log-restricted-likelihood: -2438.282
 Fixed: y ~meth + item
(Intercept)        methR         methS         item2         item3         item4
103.46310311  -0.08627451   15.61960784    5.91463879  -22.10940012    2.03820805
      item5         item6         item7         item8         item9        item10
 13.56038699   25.82329091    5.77040529    7.97908153    2.90046966   -2.42518966
     item11        item12        item13        item14        item15        item16
  0.76871795   10.82978602    8.24485168    1.91320568    1.30279930   15.29318373
     item17        item18        item19        item20        item21        item22
 -2.16371886   14.29958778   32.87490656   42.98067780   53.25328835   39.77285527
     item23        item24        item25        item26        item27        item28
 65.64110356   60.31687736   39.19365339   27.17442226   37.51905849   44.86191632
     item29        item30        item31        item32        item33        item34
115.80262665   95.16665717  -15.10771279   14.83459381   18.41497459   21.71322032
     item35        item36        item37        item38        item39        item40
 15.69685542  -12.90393540    4.21600498  105.00952450   24.86057428   30.50775559
     item41        item42        item43        item44        item45        item46
 -9.12356926   -8.19256556   17.45318264   58.61833461   -2.12382348   24.31072753
     item47        item48        item49        item50        item51        item52
 11.38115695   31.76383809   48.90518638  -11.56764476   52.58805480   -1.46339771
     item53        item54        item55        item56        item57        item58
  1.30566553   -4.32085153  -23.86901095    1.62002195    5.45942354   75.56038699
     item59        item60        item61        item62        item63        item64
 52.78027507   36.02715937   93.56376166  -12.01620175   24.34918980   36.86200739
     item65        item66        item67        item68        item69        item70
 33.61521416   54.10214235   29.71617762   10.40512379   13.26577015   17.50606826
     item71        item72        item73        item74        item75        item76
112.36689675   31.12795967   53.70166320  -19.56436116   70.43707195   75.63925308
     item77        item78        item79        item80        item81        item82
 13.62635391   16.54801525    4.65198910    7.34920879   36.64371558    5.09083945
     item83        item84        item85
  6.81873734   -1.82236623   12.46591865
```

```
 Random effects:
 Formula: ~meth - 1 | item
 Structure: Diagonal
                 methJ          methR       methS  Residual
StdDev: 0.0003511279 0.0003482782  17.95985  5.531622
```

```
Variance function:
 Structure: Different standard deviations per stratum
 Formula: ~1 | meth
 Parameter estimates:
       J        R        S
1.000000 1.005149 1.648373
Number of Observations: 765
Number of Groups: 85
```

13

The Methcomp package for R

The purpose of the MethComp package for R is to provide computational tools to manipulate, display and analyze data from method comparison studies. Further material such as exercises, course material and latest updates of the package can be found at the package website http://www.biostat.ku.dk/~bxc/MethComp. This chapter describes core parts of the package that are not likely to change much.

13.1 Data structures

In general we are concerned with measurements by different methods, on different items (persons, samples), possibly replicated. Often such data are represented by a row of measurements for each item, with possible replicates listed either below or beside each other. This implicitly assumes that the replicate measurements listed on the same line belong together, which is not necessarily the case in all situations.

All functions in MethComp assume data to be represented in 'long' form, with one measurement on each row, and columns to indicate method, item and replicate. Specifically, we assume the following columns are available in a data frame:

- meth The measurement method. Numeric or factor.

- item Identification of item (person, sample). Numeric or factor.

Comparing Clinical Measurement Methods: A Practical Guide   Bendix Carstensen
© 2010 John Wiley & Sons, Ltd

- `repl` Replicate number. Numeric or factor.

- `y` The measurement by method `meth` on item `item`, replicate number `repl`.

There is a class, `Meth`, for this kind of data frame. A data frame is converted to a `Meth` object by using the `Meth` function on it. Objects of class `Meth` (which inherits from the class `data.frame`) have specific methods such as `summary`, `plot`, `subset` and `transform`. There are several ways of creating a data frame of class `Meth` from an existing data frame – see the documentation for the function `Meth`.

13.2   Function overview

The following is a brief overview of the functions in the `MethComp` package. The full documentation is in the help pages for the functions, and an illustration of the way they work can be obtained by referring to the help pages.

13.2.1   Graphical functions

`BA.plot` Draws a Bland–Altman plot of two methods from a data frame with method comparison data, and computes limits of agreement. The plotting is really done by a call to the function `BlandAltman`.

`BlandAltman` Draws a Bland–Altman plot and computes limits of agreement. It also computes tests of whether the slope between two methods is 1 and of constant variance, and can produce the regression of the differences on the averages.

`plot.Meth` Plots all methods against all others, both as scatter plots and as a Bland–Altman plot.

`bothlines` Adds regression lines of y on x and vice versa to a scatter plot. Optionally, the Deming regression line can be added too.

13.2.2   Data manipulating functions

make.repl Generates (or replaces) a repl column in a data frame with columns meth, item and y.

perm.repl Randomly permutes replicates within (method, item) and assigns new replicate numbers.

to.wide Transforms a data frame in the long form to the wide form where separate columns for each method are generated, with one row per (item, replicate).

to.long Reverses the result of to.wide. The function can also generate a long-form data set from a data set with different methods beside each other.

summary.Meth Tabulates items by method and number of replicates for a Meth object.

Meth.sim Simulates a data set from a method comparison experiment for given parameters for bias, exchangeability and variance component sizes.

13.2.3   Analysis functions

Deming Performs Deming regression, i.e. regression with errors in both variables.

DA.reg Regresses the differences between methods on the averages and derives approximate linear conversion equations, based on [11].

BA.est Provides estimates in the variance components model (5.2), underlying the concept of limits of agreement, and returns the bias and the variance components. Assumes constant bias between methods. Returns a MethComp object.

AltReg Provides estimates via alternating regressions in the general model (7.1). Returns estimates of mean conversion parameters and variance components. The fitting algorithm is not terribly efficient, so it is advisable to use the argument trace=T to make sure that something actually is happening. Returns a MethComp object.

MCmcmc Provides estimates via BUGS in the general model with non-constant bias. Produces an MCmcmc object, which is an mcmc.list object with some extra attributes. mcmc.list objects are handled by the coda package, so this is required when calling MCmcmc. An MCmcmc object can be used to construct a MethComp object that contains the estimated conversion equations and the estimated variance components.

The functions BA.est, AltReg and MCmcmc allow a transformation the measurement values before analysis. This transformation is returned as part of the resulting MethComp object, allowing the plot.MethComp function to report the results on the original scale of measurement.

13.2.4 Reporting functions

print.MethComp Prints a table of conversion equations and estimated variance components from a MethComp object.

plot.MethComp Plots conversion lines with prediction limits, based on a MethComp object. Will also plot limits of agreement, back-transformed if a data transformation was used.

print.MCmcmc Prints a table of conversion equations between methods analyzed, with prediction standard deviations. Also gives summaries of the posteriors for the parameters that constitute the conversion algorithms.

plot.MCmcmc Plots the conversion lines between methods with prediction limits.

post.MCmcmc Plots smoothed posterior densities for the estimates. This is primarily of interest for the variance component estimates, but it has arguments to produce the posterior distribution of the parameters of the mean conversion between methods.

check.MCmcmc Draws diagnostic plots of the traces of the chains included in an MCmcmc object.

References

[1] DG Altman. Calculating age-related reference centiles using absolute residuals. *Statistics in Medicine*, 12: 917–924, 1993.

[2] DG Altman and JM Bland. Measurement in medicine: The analysis of method comparison studies. *The Statistician*, 32: 307–317, 1983.

[3] G Atkinson and A Nevill. Comment on the use of concordance correlation to assess the agreement between two variables. *Biometrics*, 52: 775–778, 1997.

[4] HX Barnhart, MJ Haber, and LI Lin. An overview on assessing agreement with continuous measurements. *Journal of Biopharmaceutical Statistics*, 17: 529–569, 2007.

[5] HX Barnhart, AS Kosinski, and MJ Haber. Assessing individual agreement. *Journal of Biopharmaceutical Statistics*, 17: 697–719, 2007.

[6] JM Bland and DG Altman. Statistical methods for assessing agreement between two methods of clinical measurement. *Lancet*, i: 307–310, 1986.

[7] JM Bland and DG Altman. Comparing methods of measurement: why plotting difference against standard method is misleading. *Lancet*, 346: 1085–1087, 1995.

[8] JM Bland and DG Altman. Measuring agreement in method comparison studies. *Statistical Methods in Medical Research*, 8: 136–160, 1999.

[9] L Brøndsted. *Quantification of agreement*. PhD thesis, Department of Biostatistics, University of Copenhagen, 2002.

[10] B Carstensen. Comparing and predicting between several methods of measurement. *Biostatistics*, 5(3): 399–413, 2004.

[11] B. Carstensen. Comparing methods of measurement: Extending the LoA by regression. *Statistics in Medicine*, 29: 401–410, 2010.

[12] B Carstensen, J Lindström, J Sundvall, K Borch-Johnsen, J Tuomilehto, and the DPS Study Group. Measurement of blood glucose: Comparison between different types of specimens. *Annals of Clinical Biochemistry*, 45(2): 140–148, 2008.

[13] B Carstensen, J Simpson, and LC Gurrin. Statistical models for assessing agreement in method comparison studies with replicate measurements. *International Journal of Biostatistics*, 4(1): Article 16, 2008.

[14] S Colagiuri, A Sandbæk, B Carstensen, J Christensen, C Glümer, T Lauritzen, and K Borch-Johnsen. Comparability of venous and capillary glucose measurements in blood. *Diabetic Medicine*, 20(11): 953–956, 2003.

[15] G Dunn. *Statistical Evaluation of Measurement Errors. Design and Analysis of Reliability Studies* (2nd edn). Arnold, 2004.

[16] Food and Drug Administration (FDA). Guidance for industry: Statistical approaches to establishing bioequivalence. Technical report, FDA, 2001, http://www.fda.gov/cder/guidance/3616fnl.pdf.

[17] International Organization for Standardization, *Accuracy (trueness and precision) of measurement methods and results – Part 2: Basic method for the determination of repeatability and reproducibility of a standard measurement method*, ISO 5725-2: 1994, www.iso.org.

[18] LI Lin. A concordance correlation coefficient to evaluate reproducibility. *Biometrics*, 45: 255–268, 1989.

[19] LI Lin. Total deviation index for measuring individual agreement with applications in laboratory performance and bioequivalence. *Statistics in Medicine*, 19: 255–270, 2000.

[20] J Shao and B Zong. Assessing the agreement between two quantitative assays with repeated measurements. *Journal of Biopharmaceutical Statistics*, 14(1): 201–214, 2004.

Index

Statistics in Practice

Human and Biological Sciences

Berger – Selection Bias and Covariate Imbalances in Randomized Clinical Trials

Berger and Wong – An Introduction to Optimal Designs for Social and Biomedical Research

Brown and Prescott – Applied Mixed Models in Medicine, Second Edition

Carstensen – Comparing Clinical Measurement Methods

Chevret (Ed) – Statistical Methods for Dose-Finding Experiments

Ellenberg, Fleming and DeMets – Data Monitoring Committees in Clinical Trials: A Practical Perspective

Hauschke, Steinijans & Pigeot – Bioequivalence Studies in Drug Development: Methods and Applications

Lawson, Browne and Vidal Rodeiro – Disease Mapping with WinBUGS and MLwiN

Lesaffre, Feine, Leroux & Declerck – Statistical and Methodological Aspects of Oral Health Research

Lui – Statistical Estimation of Epidemiological Risk

Marubini and Valsecchi – Analysing Survival Data from Clinical Trials and Observation Studies

Molenberghs and Kenward – Missing Data in Clinical Studies

O'Hagan, Buck, Daneshkhah, Eiser, Garthwaite, Jenkinson, Oakley & Rakow – Uncertain Judgements: Eliciting Expert's Probabilities

Parmigiani – Modeling in Medical Decision Making: A Bayesian Approach

Pintilie – Competing Risks: A Practical Perspective

Senn – Cross-over Trials in Clinical Research, Second Edition

Senn – Statistical Issues in Drug Development, Second Edition

Spiegelhalter, Abrams and Myles – Bayesian Approaches to Clinical Trials and Health-Care Evaluation

Walters – Quality of Life Outcomes in Clinical Trials and Health-Care Evaluation

Whitehead – Design and Analysis of Sequential Clinical Trials, Revised Second Edition
Whitehead – Meta-Analysis of Controlled Clinical Trials
Willan and Briggs – Statistical Analysis of Cost Effectiveness Data
Winkel and Zhang – Statistical Development of Quality in Medicine

Earth and Environmental Sciences

Buck, Cavanagh and Litton – Bayesian Approach to Interpreting Archaeological Data
Glasbey and Horgan – Image Analysis in the Biological Sciences
Helsel – Nondetects and Data Analysis: Statistics for Censored Environmental Data
Illian, Penttinen, Stoyan, H and Stoyan D–Statistical Analysis and Modelling of Spatial Point Patterns
McBride – Using Statistical Methods for Water Quality Management
Webster and Oliver – Geostatistics for Environmental Scientists, Second Edition
Wymer (Ed) – Statistical Framework for Recreational Water Quality Criteria and Monitoring

Industry, Commerce and Finance

Aitken – Statistics and the Evaluation of Evidence for Forensic Scientists, Second Edition
Balding – Weight-of-evidence for Forensic DNA Profiles
Brandimarte – Numerical Methods in Finance and Economics: A MATLAB-Based Introduction, Second Edition
Brandimarte and Zotteri – Introduction to Distribution Logistics
Chan – Simulation Techniques in Financial Risk Management
Coleman, Greenfield, Stewardson and Montgomery (Eds) – Statistical Practice in Business and Industry
Frisen (Ed) – Financial Surveillance
Fung and Hu – Statistical DNA Forensics
Gusti Ngurah Agung – Time Series Data Analysis Using EViews
Jank and Shmueli (Ed.) – Statistical Methods in e-Commerce Research

Lehtonen and Pahkinen – Practical Methods for Design and Analysis of Complex Surveys, Second Edition

Ohser and Mücklich – Statistical Analysis of Microstructures in Materials Science

Pourret, Naim & Marcot (Eds) – Bayesian Networks: A Practical Guide to Applications

Taroni, Aitken, Garbolino and Biedermann – Bayesian Networks and Probabilistic Inference in Forensic Science

Taroni, Bozza, Biedermann, Garbolino and Aitken – Data Analysis in Forensic Science